EARL MINDELL'S
PILL BIBLE

To THE GROSSMAN'S

STAY HEALTHY,

Love;

Earl

By Earl Mindell

Earl Mindell's Vitamin Bible
Earl Mindell's Vitamin Bible for Your Kids
Earl Mindell's Pill Bible

EARL MINDELL'S PILL BIBLE

Earl L. Mindell, R.Ph., Ph.D.

BANTAM BOOKS
TORONTO · NEW YORK · LONDON · SYDNEY

AN IMPORTANT NOTE TO ALL READERS OF THIS BOOK

The regimens throughout this book are recommendations, not prescriptions, and are not intended as medical advice, nor are they intended to replace any specific instructions or warnings given to you by your doctor or a particular product's information sheet.

EARL MINDELL'S PILL BIBLE

A Bantam Book / March 1984

All rights reserved.
Copyright © 1984 by Earl Mindell and Hester Mundis.
This book may not be reproduced in whole or in part, by
mimeograph or any other means, without permission.
For information address: Bantam Books, Inc.

Library of Congress Cataloging in Publication Data

Mindell, Earl.
  Earl Mindell's Pill bible.

  Bibliography: p.
  Includes index.
  1. Drugs—Popular works. 2. Pharmacology—Popular
works. I. Title. II. Title: Pill bible.
RM301.15.M56 1984   615.1   83-24344
ISBN 0-553-34064-6 (pbk.)

Published simultaneously in the United States and Canada

Bantam Books are published by Bantam Books, Inc. Its trade-
mark, consisting of the words "Bantam Books" and the
portrayal of a rooster, is Registered in the United States
Patent and Trademark Office and in other countries. Marca
Registrada. Bantam Books, Inc., 666 Fifth Avenue, New York,
New York 10103.

PRINTED IN THE UNITED STATES OF AMERICA

S   0 9 8 7 6 5 4 3 2 1

*This book is dedicated to Gail,
Alanna, Evan, my parents and families,
my friends and associates, and to the
health and happiness of people everywhere.*

Contents

Part One
TAKE YOUR MEDICINE

Part Two
ABECEDARY OF PILLS AND POTIONS

Part Three
MEALS AND MEDICINES

Part Four
IT TAKES ALL KINDS

Part Five
SPECIAL FOR SENIOR CITIZENS

Preface

Having been a registered pharmacist and a nutritionist for over fifteen years, I have come to realize that there is a big difference between *getting* well and *feeling* well—and I have discovered that there doesn't have to be!

I made this discovery after the publication of my first book, *The Vitamin Bible*, when—in touring and lecturing on preventive medicine and nutrition—I found that most people considered vitamins and drugs natural enemies and felt compelled to be totally committed to one or the other. Now, I am a confirmed advocate of the amazing curative properties of natural foods and vitamins, and I still believe that far too many drugs are prescribed and taken unnecessarily. But I also believe that drugs and medicines can and do cure a variety of illnesses that cannot at present be combated effectively any other way. The point is, though vitamins and drugs perform different functions for different purposes, they are not—and need not be—mutually exclusive. In fact, by fully understanding the scope and actions of both, anyone, I'm convinced, can maximize the potential for optimal health, which is why this book was written.

Upon looking over the numerous drug dictionaries on the market, I was struck by the fact that almost all of them ignored nutrition and dealt with drugs in the abstract (and technically at that!), instead of with individuals and their use of medications and foods in everyday life. Because of this, and because I know how many millions of people are taking drugs in one form or another, I felt that there was a great need for an easy-to-understand guide to what I call pharmaceutical nutrition— a way to feel well while getting well.

People often don't realize that the same drug can behave differently in different individuals. A person's age, weight, particular body chemistry, general health, and sex can and do affect the way medicines work. For example, the antibiotic that cures your bronchitis could harm your grandfather or your child—even if he or she has the same disease! Drugs are substances that do not occur in the body naturally, so, like waste products, they are gradually eliminated. But if cleansing organs like the kidneys or liver aren't functioning properly, or aren't completely mature, even seemingly harmless over-the-counter (OTC) medicines can build up in the system to a dangerous and unwanted degree.

What must be kept in mind is that pills are not "sure shot" cures. You can't *aim* a drug at an inflamed bronchial tube and expect that the rest of your body will remain untouched. Drugs are not unlike railroad trains traveling along certain tracks. You might want to just go from New York to California, and Peoria, let's say, is the last place in the world you want to see, but if it's on the route, like it or not, you do. It's sort of a necessary "side effect" of the trip.

In *The Pill Bible* I've attempted to design a practical, home-reference handbook that explains why one good pill doesn't necessarily deserve another and how natural foods and supplements can actually replace many medicines as well as help them work more effectively and alleviate side effects. It's a book that answers those questions you never thought to ask your doctor or pharmacist, and it provides you with information that they might never have thought to give you. By incorporating knowledge of the basic functions, contraindications, interactions, and side effects of hundreds of prescription and OTC drugs with an understanding of natural alternatives, potentiating and debilitating foods, vitamins, and energy-enhancing dietary regimens, you and your family will have a solid groundwork for regaining and maintaining vitality and a healthy enjoyment of life.

The book is divided into numbered, easy-to-find sections that are cross-referenced, so that you can quickly locate all information pertaining to your medication. And because drugs are often prescribed for different purposes for different people, I've tried to personalize the book as much as possible by dealing separately with women, children, senior citizens, dieters, diabetics, alcoholics, smokers, and many others.

To help you identify drugs, brand names throughout are printed in full caps. Generic names are printed in upper and lower case.

My recommendations in all instances are not meant to be prescriptive; they are offered only as suggestions, which should be discussed with your doctor. Needless to say, no book is a substitute for professional care.

My greatest hope is that this book will bridge the gap between vitamins and drugs, and enable you under any circumstances to make the most of the information gathered herein and use it to the best and healthiest of advantages for a long time to come.

Dr. Earl L. Mindell

Acknowledgments

I wish to express my deep and lasting appreciation to my many friends and colleagues who have assisted me in the preparation of this book, especially J. Kenny, Ph.D., Linus Pauling, Ph.D., Harold Segal, Ph.D., Robert Mendelson, M.D., Arnold Fox, M.D., Gershon Lesser, M.D., David Velkoff, M.D., Rory Jaffe, M.D., Bernard Bubman, R.Ph., Mel Rich, R.Ph., Sal Messineo, R.Ph., William Epstein, R.Ph., Barbara Epstein, R.N., Peter Mallory, and Hester Mundis.

I would also like to thank the International College of Applied Nutrition, the Nutrition Foundation, the International Academy of Preventative Medicine, the American Dietetic Association, the American Pharmaceutical Association, the National Academy of Sciences, the American Heart Association, the American Diabetes Association, the Arthritis Foundation, the Society for Nutrition Education, the New York Division of Substance Abuse Services, Roche Chemical Division-Vitamin Communications, the Upjohn Company, the U.S. Department of Health and Human Services; Betty Haskins, Judy Beal, Susan Towlson, Herman E. Gordon, Ron VanWarmer, and Richard Curtis, whose cooperation, resources, and enthusiastic assistance were indispensable in making this project a reality.

The desire to take medicine is perhaps
the greatest feature which distinguishes
man from animals.

Sir William Osler

Part One

TAKE YOUR MEDICINE

Chapter I

What the Doctor Ordered

1. Why certain drugs require prescriptions

> Any medication that can cause harmful side effects when taken in *regular* doses requires an Rx.

The difference between over-the-counter (OTC) medications and those that require a doctor's or dentist's written prescription is allegedly consumer safety. According to Federal Drug Administration (FDA) law, any medication that can cause harmful side effects when taken in regular doses requires an Rx. All OTC medicines, which are for the relief of symptoms only and not to be recognized as a cure, have been deemed safe if taken as directed, and are required to print warnings and contraindications clearly on the product package.

2. Who controls "controlled substances"?

The Food and Drug Administration (FDA) has classified drugs according to their potential for abuse (excessive or improper use), and the Justice Department's Drug Enforcement

Administration sees that the rules governing these classifications are adhered to.

Drugs that are deemed "controlled substances" are divided into categories (Schedules I, II, III, IV, and V), prescriptions for them are limited in duration (as well as to the number of refills), and careful records are kept on their production and distribution.

SCHEDULE I DRUGS

These drugs are basically illegal. They have either no legitimate medical use or their potential for legitimate medical use is still under investigation and not yet fully recognized (as in the case of marijuana use to alleviate the side effects of chemotherapy).

Some examples are:

Heroin	Marijuana
LSD	Peyote
Mescaline	Psilocybin
Hashish	Tetrahydrocannabinol (THC)
Ketobemidone	Levomoramide
Racemoramide	Benzylmorphine
Dihydromorphine	Nicocodeine

SCHEDULE II DRUGS

Medications in this class are essentially narcotic, stimulant, and depressant drugs. Though they have legitimate medical uses, they cannot be prescribed by a doctor (or other authorized registered practitioner) over the phone except in cases of emergency because of their high abuse potential, particularly in the areas of psychological and physical dependence. (See section 85.)

Some examples are:

Opium	Morphine
Codeine	Hydromorphone
Methadone (DOLOPHINE)	(DILAUDID)
Meperidine (DEMEROL)	Cocaine

Oxycodone (PERCODAN)
Oxymorphone
    (NUMORPHAN)
Methamphetamine
    (DESOXYN)
Methylphenidate
    (RITALIN)
Pentobarbital
    (NEMBUTAL)
Methaqualone
    (QUAALUDE)
Diphenoxylate

Anileridine (LERITINE)
Amphetamine
    (DEXEDRINE)
Phenmetrazine
    (PRELUDIN)
Amobarbital (AMYTAL)

SCHEDULE III DRUGS

These drugs have less abuse potential than those in Schedules I and II. Primarily the category includes compounds that contain limited quantities of certain narcotic and non-narcotic drugs, and they can be prescribed over the telephone.
Some examples are:

Glutethimide (DORIDEN)
Chlorphentermine
    (PRE-SATE)
Mazindol (SANOREX)
Paregoric
Secobarbital
    (SECONAL, TUINAL)

Methyprylon (NOLUDAR)
Benzphetamine
    (DIDREX)
Clortermine (VORANIL)
Phendimetrazine
    (PHENAZINE)

SCHEDULE IV DRUGS

These drugs have a lower abuse potential than those in Schedule III, though they are among the most widely prescribed in the U.S.
Some examples are:

Barbital
Methylphenobarbital
Chloral hydrate
Ethinamate (VALMID)

Phenobarbital
Ethchlorvynol (PLACIDYL)
Meprobamate
    (EQUANIL, MILTOWN)

Paraldehyde
Fenfluramine
  (PONDIMIN)
Phentermine (IONAMIN)
Diazepam (VALIUM)
Clorazepate (TRANXENE)
Clonazepam (CLONOPIN)
Lorazepam (ATIVAN)
Propoxyphene
  hydrochloride
  (DARVON)

Methohexital
  (BREVITAL SODIUM)
Diethylpropion
  (TENUATE)
Chlordiazepoxide
  (LIBRIUM)
Oxazepam (SERAX)
Flurazepam (DALMANE)
Prazepam (CENTRAX,
  VERSTRAN)
Pentazocine (TALWIN)

SCHEDULE V DRUGS

These drugs have a still lower abuse potential than those in the other classes and consist mainly of preparations containing very limited quantities of narcotic substances, primarily cough syrups and antidiarrhea medications.
Some examples are:

NOVAHISTINE DH
ROBITUSSIN A-C
TYLENOL WITH
  CODEINE ELIXIR
TRIAMINIC WITH
  CODEINE
TERPIN HYDRATE &
  CODEINE ELIXIR
NALDECON CX
  SUSPENSION

LOMOTIL
PAREPECTOLIN
AMBENYL
  EXPECTORANT

3. What is an Rx and how to read it

A prescription is a written direction by a physician, dentist, podiatrist, veterinarian (or other authorized registered practitioner) to a pharmacist for medication. It specifies the name of the drug, exact dosage, how much should be dispensed, and directions for administering it.

Though that slip you carry to the pharmacist might look like Greek to you, it's actually Latin (abbreviations), and not all that difficult to decipher.

ad lib	freely, generally pertaining to instructions for refilling Rx
a.c.	before meals
b.i.d.	twice a day
co., comp.	compound
d.	per day
dur. dol.	while the pain lasts
e.m.p.	as prescribed
gr.	grain, grains (1 grain = approximately 65 mg.)
gtt.	drops
h.s.	at bedtime
mg	milligrams
o.d.	every day
O.D.	in right eye
O.S.	in left eye
O.U.	in each eye
p.c.	after meals
p.r.n.	as needed
pro us. ext.	for external use
q.h., q.2 h., etc.	every hour, every two hours, etc.
q.s.	as much as necessary
sig.	label
s.o.s.	if necessary
stat.	immediately
t.i.d.	three times a day
ut dict.	as directed

Before leaving the pharmacy, check the label on the prescription you're taking home. Make sure it lists these six things:

1. The date
2. Patient's name (and, as an additional safety measure, address)
3. Doctor's name
4. Name of drug (generic and/or trade)
5. Instructions for use
6. Prescription number

Also, because it is not a worldwide—or even nationwide—requirement, I advise you to ask your physician to direct the pharmacist to include on the label the strength of the medication, the amount (number of pills, ounces, etc.), and the expiration date (when the medication might no longer be effective, and even harmful). (See section 12.) This information could actually mean the difference between life and death if you or anyone else should take an overdose of the medication.

4. Generic vs. name brands

Consumers continue to be confused by the constant controversies over generic vs. name brand drugs. To most people, a generic drug is the same as a name brand drug, only more difficult to pronounce and cheaper. Well, this is not untrue, but it's not entirely true either.

> Just because your doctor writes a generic prescription doesn't necessarily mean you'll be paying less.

But if you understand the process involved in bringing a new drug to market, you'll be in a much better position to evaluate and discuss your prescription with your physician and your pharmacist, keeping your pocketbook in mind.

BIRTH OF A PRESCRIPTION DRUG

- While a drug is undergoing clinical tests and investigation, it gets a number; and the United States Adopted Names Council gives it a *generic* name.
- The chemical formulation of the drug usually becomes the basis of the generic name.
- When the FDA declares the drug safe and effective, the pharmaceutical company can give its product a catchy, easily memorable *brand name*, which is then registered and trademarked.
- This new drug holds exclusive patent rights for seventeen years, which means rival firms may not duplicate it. Therefore, a prescription written for its generic name might cost just as much as one for its brand name.

- After seventeen years, other companies may manufacture the same drug, but under different *brand* names.

The only advantage of brand name drugs over generic drugs is, to my mind, a questionable one: that of *bioavailability*. This refers to the amount of active medication that actually reaches the bloodstream and the time it takes to do its job. Because different drug companies do use different stabilizers and binders in their manufacturing process, some virtually identical drugs made by different manufacturers will have varying bioavailability. But the degrees of bioavailability are rarely worth the difference in price.

My advice: Shop around for a good well-stocked pharmacy, and always ask your physician to prescribe generically, or at least indicate that a generic product can be substituted. A pharmacist cannot sell you a generic product if your doctor has specified a name brand. But—even when you have a generic prescription—if your pharmacy carries the product only in a high-priced name brand, that's what you're going to get—and pay for!

5. Be aware of the name game

A rose by any other name might smell just as sweet, but a drug by any other name can cost more money and be just as effective—or *ineffective*—in treating your illness.

For example, a patient whose illness is not responding to treatment with Lederle's ACHROMYCIN V won't fare any better with Squibb's SUMYCIN or Bristol's TETREX or Upjohn's PANMYCIN. They're all the same antibiotic *tetracycline*!

Beecham Lab's AMOXIL and Roche's LAROTID might sound different, but they're both *amoxicillin* and they perform identical functions. The same holds true for dozens and dozens of other prescription medicines.

To be sure that the medicine you're taking now is or isn't the same as the one you were taking before, check the brand and generic name listings in sections 32–52.

6. Any questions about Chapter I?

Do all prescription drugs have to have those awful, hard-to-open, "child-resistant" caps?

It is a law (and a good one, since childhood poisonings have already been cut in half), but if you have no children in your home and would prefer an easier to open container, you can just file a permission slip with your pharmacist, and you can get your prescription drugs with an easier opening lid.

When doctors phone prescriptions into pharmacies, how do pharmacists know that they're really doctors (or dentists)?

Doctors (and dentists) have a registry number from the government, a DEA (Drug Enforcement Agency) number, which they must give to the pharmacist when ordering a prescription drug for a patient.

Is the PDR [Physicians' Desk Reference] the book that will tell me everything about my medication?

The PDR, which is published annually by Medical Economics Company, Inc., has fairly complete information on over 2,000 drugs. But this information is essentially technical, written for professionals such as doctors and pharmacists, and the entries are supplied and paid for by the pharmaceutical houses themselves. All the information, though, is in accordance with the current FDA labeling requirements for the drugs.

But, as I said, the book is not designed for the layperson. Without a technical background in the field, you'd probably be better off asking your pharmacist or doctor what you want to know about your medication, or checking your drug out in one of the books in this book's Bibliography which has been written in language and terms that the general public can understand.

Do you have any idea when drugs like VALIUM and DALMANE will be available generically?

The patent for VALIUM (*diazepam*) will expire in 1985, and the one for DALMANE (*flurazepam*) in 1989. At that time, other companies may manufacture the drug under other brand names, and if your doctor prescribes the drugs generically, you'll probably be able to get them for less money (assuming your pharmacist will stock the less expensive brands).

Other drugs soon to be available from competing manufacturers are INDERAL (1984), ALDOMET (1984), CLINORIL (1989), NAPROSYN (1989), KEFLEX (1987), DIABINESE (1984), LOPRESSOR (1988), CLEOCIN (1986), ALDORIL (1984), MINIPRESS (1987), TIMOPTIC (1988), ZYLOPRIM (1986), TRANXENE (1987), TRIAVIL (1985), HALDOL (1986), ATIVAN (1986), NALFON (1988), and SINEQUAN (1987).

Chapter II

At the Pharmacy

7. What pharmacists do and don't know about drugs

> Your pharmacist usually knows more than your physician about the drug you're taking!

Pharmacists, aside from dispensing prescription medicines and giving advice on the use of over-the-counter preparations, are the people who know the most about drugs.

- Pharmacists are specifically trained in pharmacology and therefore are the people who best understand the use, composition, and effect of drugs as well as how they are tested for strength and purity. (Doctors do not have as extensive training in pharmacology.)
- Most pharmacists do maintain patient medication profiles, which list the drugs you're taking, and can alert you and your doctor to possible dangerous interactions.
- Pharmacists can advise physicians on the proper selection and use of new medicines.
- Pharmacists are generally well informed on the medicines they stock and can explain how a drug is to be

taken, what side effects can be expected, what toxicities you should be aware of, when the drug is contraindicated, and what precautions you should take while on the medication.

Pharmacists can suggest and advise you of the advantages and disadvantages of OTC medicines.

BUT

- Pharmacists are *not* doctors and are not in a position to discuss or dispute a doctor's diagnosis and/or the ramifications of diseases.
- Pharmacists cannot prescribe medicines.

8. Questions to ask when buying medicines

If something is going into—or onto—your body, you should know what that something is. You should also know what it can do—or what it *might* do.

The following is a list of questions that you should know the answers to before leaving a pharmacy with any drug or medication:

- What is the name, dosage, and function of the drug?
- How often should it be taken or applied? (Does four times a day mean every six hours; or morning, noon, suppertime, and bedtime?)
- Should it be taken with or without food? Before or after meals?
- Can it be taken with milk? Juice? Protein?
- Are there any food, vitamin, or other medicines that I should not have while on this medication?
- What side effects should I be aware of?
- Does smoking affect the medication? Does alcohol? How?
- What should I do if I miss a dose?
- When should I expect to feel or see results from the medication?
- How long should I take the medicine?

- How should the medicine be stored?
- Have I—according to your records—taken a similar drug before?

These questions should be asked about *all* medications, whether they are prescription or OTC, systemic (taken internally) or topical (applied externally). (A simple OTC antibiotic ointment is capable of causing more complications than the wound it's applied to, if you're unaware that the ointment has the potential for uncomfortable allergic side effects.)

Caution: Most OTC drugs, which are legally considered reasonably safe for use by the public for minor illnesses without consulting a physician, are not specifically intended to be used during pregnancy or lactation. Because of this, all pregnant and nursing mothers *should definitely consult the pharmacist before taking any OTC medication.* (See section 68.)

9. How long will it keep?

Nothing lasts forever—least of all medicines. Any medication you buy—whether it is an over-the-counter preparation or a prescription drug—should have an expiration date on the package or label.

An expiration date is the time until which the drug will remain stable and effective when stored under recommended conditions.

A safe rule of thumb for prescription medicines, which usually don't carry an expiration date, is two weeks for liquid medications that require refrigeration (you can ask your pharmacist about the effective shelf life of cough medicines and tonics, which have longer medicinal staying powers) and approximately two years for pills or capsules.

10. How to store your medicines

Why medicine cabinets were designed to fit into bathrooms is beyond me. The worst place to store pills and capsules is in a place where there is constant moisture and heat.

> The worst place to keep your medicines can be
> the bathroom medicine cabinet!

Pills and capsules should be stored in a cool dry place and
out of direct bright light or sunlight. (Needless to say—or
perhaps *not* needless to say—they should also be kept out of the
reach of children.) Pills that are exposed to moisture have a
tendency to disintegrate and lose potency. Always keep the top
or cover of a pill bottle tightly closed. Give one unclosed box of
capsules one humid day, and you'll find yourself with something that looks like a model of Mars with mumps.

Most liquid antibiotics should be stored in the refrigerator.
This preserves the bacteria-fighting effectiveness of the medicine.
But refrigeration does *not* mean freezing. Freezing can change
the molecular structure of the medicine and undermine its
healing properties.

Anal and vaginal suppositories are usually stored in a very
cool place or the refrigerator to prevent melting and facilitate
insertion.

In all cases, check with your pharmacist on the proper
method of storage for any medicines you buy.

11. How to tell if your medicine has "spoiled"

1. Check expiration date.
2. Solutions and liquids: Odor should not change; color
   and taste should not be different from what they were
   originally.
3. Pills and tablets: They should retain their original size,
   weight, and color. Chips, cracks, and splits in pills and
   tablets are a sign of decay. Any unusual odor is also a
   sign of deterioration.
4. Gelatin capsules: Capsule shells that have softened and
   stick together, or have hardened and crack under slight
   pressure have "spoiled."
5. Ointments: A change in consistency, such as the ointment becoming too hard or too soft, or "bleeding"—which
   is a liquid running from the tube—is a sign of decay.

12. What outdated medicines can harm you

Most outdated medicines merely lose their effectiveness if kept too long, but the harm in this is that you're not getting the medicine you need when you need it. For example, using an old bottle of liquid antibiotic for a child's new strep infection can be dangerous, because the strep infection is not, in fact, being treated at all!

Some cough medicines, if kept beyond their expiration date, become more potent—but not necessarily therapeutically so. In other words, they become capable of producing stronger side effects without equivalent benefits.

There are instances, though, where a drug may become harmful due to chemical changes. Some antibiotics, for instance, if used long after their expiration date, can cause serious liver and kidney damage.

13. Any questions about Chapter II?

In liquid medicines, what is the difference between an "elixir" and a "tincture"?
None, really. Both simply mean that the drug itself is carried in an alcohol solution.

Why don't all prescription drugs that you get at the pharmacy come with those patient package inserts that doctors get with their samples?
There has been a lot of lobbying for and against this. The pharmaceutical houses and the pharmacists don't want to incur the extra expenses involved in dispensing the inserts with all individual prescriptions. Though supporters of the movement feel that these inserts would be an important tool for educating the consumer about his or her medication, detractors feel that the inserts are too technical to be of any real value, and might even be dangerously misunderstood. In some states, though, patient package inserts are required by law for certain medications, specifically hormones and birth control pills.

Does a pharmacist have to fill a doctor's prescription?
No he doesn't, especially not if he suspects that the pre-

scription was issued for other than legitimate medical purposes. In fact, if the pharmacist chooses to "look the other way" and fills a prescription that he or she knows is dubiously legitimate, the pharmacist as well as the issuing physician can be prosecuted under the law.

Are there any OTC drugs that you feel pharmacists should warn people about, but usually don't?

Lots. But I think that buyers of antihistamines and decongestants, which are among the most widely purchased OTC products, should be made aware of the fact that these medications can cause drowsiness, impair driving ability, and be dangerous if used while operating machinery. (And they can cause double trouble if combined with alcohol.) Warnings are printed on the packages, but most people don't take the time to read them. I feel that pharmacists should stress this caution since so many people feel that any drug sold over the counter has to be safe.

Chapter III

Only as Directed

14. Tell the doctor about your diet before filling that Rx

Unless it is applicable to your illness, most doctors don't ask you about your diet before handing you a prescription, so it's up to you to tell them. I say this because most people are unaware of the effects that their eating habits can have on their medications—and often the need for them!

FOODS FOR THOUGHT

- If you're a regular eater of large amounts of raw cabbage, that could be the reason for your underactive thyroid production and/or your iodine deficiency.
- Salads are great sources of vitamins and minerals, but if you're an excessive eater of raw leafy vegetables—especially cauliflower, spinach, and brussels sprouts—you may reverse the anticoagulant activity of such blood-thinning medications as COUMADIN, DICUMAROL, and HEPARIN among others (as well as the blood-thinning properties of OTC *aspirin*).
- Brewer's yeast, wheat germ, avocado, beans, liver, and heart are some prime sources of vitamin B_6, but vitamin

B_6 should not be taken by anyone under *levodopa* treatment for Parkinson's disease—and a diet very high in the above-mentioned foods could reduce the effects of your medication. (Merck Sharp & Dohme's SINEMET is a combination of *levodopa* and *carbidopa*, and the *carbidopa* prevents the reversal of effects caused by vitamin B_6, pyridoxine. Since vitamin B_6 helps alleviate nausea—often caused by *levodopa* treatments—you might want to ask your doctor about this drug.)

- If you're a heavy coffee or tea drinker, a chocolate lover, a cola addict (diet or regular), or all of the above, your consumption of caffeine could be the cause of your iron deficiency anemia.
- If you're on a low-fat or no-fat diet and you want to clear up a fungus infection quickly, you might have a problem if you don't mention this to the doctor, who'll probably prescribe *griseofulvin* (FULVICIN, GRIFULVIN V, GRISACTIN), which is absorbed faster when taken with or after high-fat meals.
- Most important! Be sure to tell your doctor about any other medicine—prescription or OTC—that you take. Also, let your doctor know if you smoke (see sections 161–166) or drink (See Sections 156–160).

15. Dangers in altering prescribed dosages

The effectiveness of a drug depends on four things:
1. The type of drug
2. The amount you take
3. How often you take it and what you take it with
4. For how long a period you take it

All drugs do *not* work in—or on—your body in the same way. Some medications must be taken for several weeks before the patient begins to feel better; for instance, tricyclic antidepressants (ELAVIL, NORPRAMIN, SINEQUAN, TOFRANIL, etc.). (See section 35.)

BUT KEEP IN MIND

- Doubling up on medication will *not* necessarily bring results any faster. In fact, doing so can seriously jeopardize your health.
- Taking less than your prescribed dosage can be dangerous. (Some people feel that by not finishing their prescribed dosage they're heroes, or that they are saving money by not having to refill the prescription as soon, or that by extending the period of treatment they'll be more effectively cured. All of these assumptions are hazardously false. For instance, taking an antibiotic only until you feel well, instead of for the full prescribed treatment, can not only cause the infection to recur but allow the invading organism to build up a tolerance to the antibiotic and therefore require more to wipe out the same infection.)
- Medicines should be given only to the person for whom they were prescribed. (The *tetracycline* that cured your 15-year-old's strep infection could permanently damage your 6-year-old's teeth.)

All medicines vary in potency, meaning it takes a smaller amount of some drugs to produce a desired effect than it does others.

If you divide doses into levels, there are *subthreshold doses*, *threshold doses*, and *ceiling doses*. Doses that produce no effect at all are called *subthreshold doses*. A *threshold dose* is the amount necessary for a drug to have any effect at all. *Ceiling doses* are those at which the drug no longer produces any further desired effect (and in fact can produce just the opposite).

An easy example is *aspirin*. An adult with a headache needs at least 200 mg. of *aspirin* to get any relief, because this is that drug's *threshold dose* for headache pain. (The average *aspirin* tablet contains 325 mg. of *aspirin*.) But the *ceiling dose* for this is 975 mg. (three tablets), which means that taking more than three tablets at one time for a headache (arthritis pain *threshold* and *ceiling doses* are higher) will produce no further relief—and will probably produce undesirable side effects.

In other words, doctors prescribe specific drugs in specific doses for specific reasons, and it's how much and how often and how long a drug is taken that produce desired results—not just the drug itself!

16. How long it takes drugs to be effective

Drugs reach their peak effect in your system at different times, depending on the type of drug, how it is administered, and your body's physical condition.

- Almost any drug you take orally becomes effective more rapidly if taken on an empty stomach.
- Pills generally take between 15 and 45 minutes (on an empty stomach) to reach peak effect; liquids reach peak effect in a shorter time, about 10 to 15 minutes.
- Some medications, specifically antifungals such as *griseofulvin*, are taken with meals to lessen stomach upset, but reach their peak effect faster if those meals are high in fat.
- Sublingual tablets (those placed under the tongue), such as antianginals (see section 46) and *ergotamine tartrate* medications for migraine headaches (ERGOMAR, ERGOSTAT, among others), are absorbed through the sublingual mucous membranes and become effective in one to three minutes.
- Time-release pills carry the medication in tiny pills, placed in a capsule, that dissolve at different rates in your stomach and intestine. This, in theory, keeps the drug working at a steadier rate for a longer amount of time. But the *United States Pharmocopeia* (USP) and the *National Formulary* (NF) have found spansules not acceptable because of their variable absorption time and course of action. ORNADE, a common cold and nasal-congestion spansule, and COMBID SPANSULES, a medication for irritable bowel, ulcers, and functional diarrhea, are among many prescription drugs found too unpredictable to provide steady 10 or 12 hours of drug availability.
- Intravenous injection—injecting the drug directly into the vein—puts the medication directly into the bloodstream. This type of administration is used when it's

essential to obtain drug effects within one to three minutes. Potent pain-killers, such as *morphine* and *nalbuphine hydrochloride* (NUBAIN), are usually administered in this fashion. Also, when there is severe infection, antibiotics such as *penicillin G sodium* are intravenously injected.

- Subcutaneous injections, those where the medicine is injected under the skin, are used when rapid onset of effects is necessary and/or when the medicine cannot—as in the case of most insulin (MONOTARD, ACTRAPID, etc.)—be taken by mouth because it is destroyed by stomach acids. Effects of subcutaneous injections are realized in one to three minutes.

- Intramuscular injections are used also for drugs requiring a relatively rapid onset or those that cannot be absorbed through the stomach. Medication is administered in this fashion because it is absorbed more slowly into the bloodstream but remains in the system for a longer period of time.

- Ordinarily, the *longer it takes* for a drug to become effective in the body, the *longer it remains* effective in your system. Conversely, the quicker a drug takes effect, the faster it is eliminated from your system.

- Suppositories can get drugs into the bloodstream fairly rapidly because the medication in the suppository is absorbed through the mucous membrane of the lower bowel. (Effects one to five minutes)

- Inhalers also provide fast action for drugs by allowing them to be absorbed through the mucous membranes of the throat and lungs. Some antiasthma preparations, such as BECLOVENT and VANCERIL, are used this way.

17. How long drugs stay in your system

The length of time that drugs stay in your system and the length of time that they're actively performing the function for which they were prescribed are two different things.

Sometimes the body can metabolize a drug rapidly by changing its molecular structure, thereby eliminating it quickly. More often, it takes about 72 hours to eliminate a drug from the tissues.

The liver plays a major role in the detoxification and elimination of drugs, which is why doctors will usually check your liver function before putting you on any extended drug regimen. Without proper detoxification and elimination facilities in your body, serious overdoses can occur.

Many conditions can affect normal hepatic (liver) functions:
- Acute hepatitis
- Chronic hepatitis
- Cirrhosis
- Tumors
- Gilbert's syndrome (which causes changes in bilirubin metabolism affecting the normal detoxification of drugs)
- Lipoid disorders (conditions where fats accumulate in excessive quantities in the body)

If you are aware of any of these conditions, consult with your doctor before taking any prescription or OTC medication!

On the other hand, some drugs have been shown to act as direct hepatoxins (substances that adversely affect the liver), and if you're taking any of these drugs regularly, you should be aware of their potential for decreasing effective liver function.

SOME COMMON DRUGS THAT CAN ADVERSELY AFFECT LIVER FUNCTIONS

- Acetaminophen (DATRIL, LIQUIPRIN, PHENAPHEN, SK-APAP, TEMPRA, TYLENOL, TYLENOL EXTRA STRENGTH, VALADOL)
- Aspirin (in high doses) (EMPIRIN COMPOUND—which is codeine and aspirin)
- Isoniazid (INH, NYDRAZID)
- Methotrexate (MEXATE)
- Tannic acid (found in tea)
- Tetracyclines (in high doses) (ACHROMYCIN, CYCLO-PAR, PANMYCIN, RETET, ROBITET, SUMYCIN, TETRACYN)

18. Adjusting dosages for kids and the elderly

Where medicines are concerned, one size *doesn't* fit all! Size counts, as does age and physical condition.

- Drugs are prescribed for adults in varying strengths, according to the nature of the illness and body weight of the patient.
- Dosages for adults are usually calculated on the weight of the average adult male—154 pounds (70 kg.)—and reduced proportionately for patients that are physically smaller. (A 100-pound model, for instance, would need a smaller dosage of a sleeping pill than a 250-pound quarterback with the same type of insomnia.)
- Children over 12 years of age are usually considered adults in terms of medicine dosage.
- Children between the ages of 5 and 12 who are of average size can usually take a third to a half of an appropriate adult medicine. (Note: Many medications, especially those that affect the central nervous system, should not be given to children at any time unless a physician advises you to do so.)
- Infants and children under the age of five do not have fully developed internal systems, and parents should *not* give such youngsters any adult medication without the advice of a physician.
- Senior citizens over the age of 65 generally need less of a drug than the average adult. Before adjusting a dosage, check with a pharmacist or a physician to be sure you're still getting enough of the drug for it to be effective. (See section 109.)

19. How to give and take medicines

The most important things to keep in mind when giving or taking medicines are *how much, how often,* and *how.*

- A teaspoon is exactly 5 ml. (milliliters). A kitchen measuring spoon (not any old spoon you use for stirring tea), a calibrated measuring cup, or an oral syringe, which are available at most pharmacies, are the only ways to provide an accurate dose.
- Drops should be measured with a medicine dropper; the eyes are not accurate counters.
- Liquid medicines should be shaken *thoroughly*, each time, before the medicine is taken.

- Always turn the lights on and check that you have the right medicine before giving or taking it; pill bottles look very much alike in the dark.
- When taking the top off a liquid medicine, keep the inner side of the cap facing up so as not to pick up any germs on the table or sink.
- To take nose drops effectively, lie on your back and tilt your head backward. After putting the drops in each nostril, remain in the same position until the medication reaches your sinuses—about two to four minutes. (IM-PORTANT: Always clean the dropper out with water and wipe it with a tissue before placing it back in the bottle.)
- Oral aerosol inhalers, which are used often in the treatment of acute and chronic bronchial asthma, pulmonary emphysema, bronchitis, and bronchiectasis, should be handled with care and not used near an open flame. To use an oral aerosol correctly, exhale fully, shake the medication, and then place the mouthpiece between your lips. Activate the inhalation release and inhale deeply. Keep your lips closed when removing the inhaler from your mouth. (IMPORTANT: If you wear contact lenses, avoid getting any of the aerosol propellant on them.)
- Before taking ear drops, clean and dry the external ear canal with a sterile cotton applicator, then lie down with your affected ear facing upwards. While in this position, administer the medicine (which should be slightly above room temperature), and remain in the same position until the drops penetrate into the ear canal—about five minutes.
- If giving a pill or capsule to someone else, either let the patient take it from the bottle himself, or put it in a paper cup or on a spoon. *Do not* carry the medication in your hand; the moisture from your palm could soften or contaminate the drug.
- Cold water helps mask unpleasant medicine taste.
- To prevent an infant from spitting out liquid medicine, put the tip of the dropper *beside* the tongue (not on it) far back in the baby's mouth.

- For patients, especially children, who can't swallow pills, tablets can be crushed and mixed with a teaspoon of applesauce, honey, or jam.
- When mixing a liquid or powder medicine in a drink, make sure you don't give too large a drink or the patient, particularly a youngster, might not finish all the medicine.
- When giving medications with liquids, water is usually best, since there are certain drugs which should not be taken with fruit juice or milk.

DRUGS THAT SHOULD *NOT* BE TAKEN WITH FRUIT JUICE

Ampicillin	Nafcillin
Cloxacillin	Oxacillin
ERYTHROCIN	Penicillin g
Erythromycin	Penicillin vk
ILOSONE	TEGOPEN
LEDERCILLIN VK	UNIPEN

(Fruit juices promote rapid breakdown of these drugs in the stomach and decrease the medicine's antibacterial action.)

DRUGS THAT SHOULD *NOT* BE TAKEN WITH MILK

(BUT CAN BE TAKEN WITH FRUIT JUICE)

ACHROMYCIN	SUMYCIN
DECLOMYCIN	TERRAMYCIN
PANMYCIN	Tetracycline

(Milk and dairy products inhibit the absorption of these medicines.)

20. Any questions about Chapter III?

Is there any special trick to using decongestant sprays? I'm sure I'm doing something wrong, since I never seem to get the "long-lasting" relief they promise in the TV ads. In fact, I usually wind up feeling more stuffed up than before.

I'm not surprised. Nasal decongestants are notorious for providing short-term relief from stuffy sinuses; with extended use the nasal membranes swell even more when the drug wears off, requiring larger and more frequent doses. A vicious cycle that takes its toll on your pocketbook as well as your health. Many decongestants also contain antihistamines, such as *phenylephrine hydrochloride* and *phenylpropanolamine hydrochloride*, which act on small blood vessels to shrink nasal membranes, but they'll act on the rest of your system too (raise blood pressure, increase heart rate, stimulate the nervous system), and do virtually nothing to help a common cold.

If you're determined to use a decongestant spray, use it only for one or two days (unless, of course, otherwise directed by your physician). Clear each nasal passage before use, then bend your head forward with your chin touching your chest. Place the nozzle of the medicine bottle slightly in your nostril, squeeze firmly, and sniff in. After use, clean the nozzle of the medicine bottle with water and wipe with a clean tissue.

Personally, I'd advise you forego the decongestants and increase the citrus fruits and juices in your diet, along with green leafy vegetables. If you really want "long-lasting" relief from cold or allergy congestion, try the following supplement (adults only) regimen:

High-potency multiple vitamin with chelated minerals	2 times daily
Rose hips vitamin C	1,000 mg. 3 to 5 times daily
Vitamin A	25,000 IU 1 to 2 times daily (take for 3 days)
3 acidophilus capsules	3 times daily
Water	6 to 8 glasses daily

If I don't know how to take a medicine—I mean, whether to take it on an empty stomach or with meals—which is best?

If you're confused or in doubt and can't consult your doctor or pharmacist, you're better off taking the medication with food. It might inhibit the drug's action a bit, but it will help prevent an upset stomach.

Is there some trick for breaking tablets in half? Even when I use a sharp knife, it seems as if a lot of my pill is left in crumbs on the kitchen counter.

Most tablets that are prescribed to be broken in half are

scored and usually convexly curved to make the process easier.
Just hold the tablet with your thumbs on either side of the
score line (which should be facing you) and press down firmly.
This should work, but if you continue having difficulty, discuss
the problem with your doctor or pharmacist and find out
whether you can get the medication in a lower dosage tablet
that doesn't have to be split.

*I take vitamins every day, but I don't think of them as drugs
so I never mention them to my doctor when he prescribes a
medication. Should I?*

Vitamins aren't drugs, but they can affect drugs and you
should definitely tell your doctor which vitamins you're taking.
Vitamin C, for instance, can reduce the effectiveness of some
antipsychotic medications, such as PERMITIL and PROLIXIN.
If you're on sulfonamides, such as GANTRISIN or THIOSULFIL
FORTE, for treatment of a urinary infection, high doses of
vitamin C can, in conjunction with these drugs, cause the development of kidney stones. Also, any aspirin-containing drug can
be affected by vitamin C, which keeps the aspirin in the body
longer and could cause an unwanted buildup. Ironically, though,
aspirin robs the body of vitamin C. If you're taking aspirin or
an aspirin-containing drug, supplements of vitamin C are
recommended, but check with your doctor to make sure the
dosage won't adversely affect your medication. Keep in mind,
too, that large doses of vitamin C can cause incorrect results on
urine glucose tests.

Vitamin B_6 can inhibit the effectiveness of the anti-Parkinson
disease drug *levodopa,* and too much riboflavin (Vitamin B_2)
can do the same for the anticancer drug *methotrexate* (MEXATE).

Chapter IV

Being a Drug Detective

21. Symptoms that could indicate the need for a prescription change

The reason you take medicine is to get better and feel better, but be aware that there is always an element of risk in taking drugs. Few medications bring instantaneous relief, and none are free from all side effects. You, as the patient, are the one who ultimately must judge whether the benefits—or potential benefits—outweigh the risks or adverse reactions caused by a particular drug.

> As a general rule, if after forty-eight hours on a medication you're feeling worse instead of better you're on the wrong medication.

Unfortunately, many people believe that just because a doctor prescribes a drug for them it's the *right* drug. But this isn't so. What might be the "right" drug for your illness might *not* be the right drug for you. For example, *penicillin G* might be the "right" drug to treat a strep throat infection, but if you're allergic to the drug it can be extremely dangerous, and if the microorganism (germ) has built up a tolerance to it it can be utterly ineffective.

My feeling is that if—after forty-eight hours on a medication—you're feeling worse instead of better, chances are you're on the wrong medication. (For exceptions, see special notes sections 32–52.) This is not to say that all danger signals occur in the first 48 hours; some are insidiously subtle and long-term. The thing to keep in mind is that we're all individuals with our own individual body chemistries; everyone will not respond the same way to the same drug. In fact, you might even respond differently to the same drug at different times, which is why it's important if you're taking medicines to be a drug detective. You're the one who knows best whether your medication is working properly or not.

WHEN TAKING ANY MEDICATION, INFORM YOUR DOCTOR AS SOON AS POSSIBLE IF . . .

- you begin to itch or develop a rash
- you have difficulty in swallowing
- your response to the drug seems the opposite of what it was prescribed for
- swelling or other sign of irritation not present before using medication occurs
- fever develops, when none was present before
- nausea and vomiting occur
- you find yourself becoming clumsy and unsteady
- your heart seems to be beating much faster or slower than usual
- muscle cramps become noticeable
- urination becomes difficult or frequent
- you notice a continual ringing or buzzing in your ears
- breathing becomes difficult or rapid
- you find yourself unusually depressed
- chest pain develops
- you become aware of persistent or frequent headaches
- your hands or feet become numb or develop a tingling/ burning sensation
- you notice any yellowing of your skin or eyes

- there is any swelling or puffiness of your face, hands, or feet
- your vision becomes blurred or double
- you find that you bruise or bleed easily or unusually
- you have a rapid unexplained gain or loss of weight
- severe indigestion, stomach pain, uncommon diarrhea or constipation develops
- extreme dizziness, fainting, or any type of seizure occurs

AND MOST IMPORTANT

- the condition for which you are taking the medication shows no sign of improvement.

22. What's in that medicine?

There's more to drugs than meets the eye, and much more that meets the system unseen. For instance, many doctors are now warning their patients to cut down on their consumption of caffeine, stressing its presence in coffee, tea, chocolate, and cola drinks, but they're not warning patients about the hidden presence of caffeine in dozens of frequently prescribed drugs and popularly purchased OTC medications.

> About 1,000 prescription products and approximately twice that many nonprescription drugs still contain caffeine!

A recent study by the FDA has linked caffeine to birth defects in laboratory animals, and scientists at Johns Hopkins University have shown that caffeine can interfere with DNA replication. Though former FDA Commissioner Jere Goyan has stressed that there is no "conclusive evidence" yet that caffeine has ever caused a birth defect in a human being, he nevertheless advises pregnant women to avoid caffeine-containing foods and drugs, or use them sparingly. With about 2,000 OTC and 1,000 prescription products still containing the substance, it's wise to know just how much of the drug (*which caffeine is*) you're getting with your medicine.

CAFFEINE-PLENTY DRUGS

Prescription	*Caffeine content in milligrams per pill*
CAFERGOT TABLETS	100 mg.
DARVON COMPOUND	32.4 mg.
FIORINAL TABLETS or CAPSULES	40 mg.
MIGRALAM CAPSULES	100 mg.
MIGRAL TABLETS	50 mg.
SOMA COMPOUND	32 mg.

Nonprescription

ANACIN ANALGESIC TABLETS	32 mg.
ANACIN MAXIMUM STRENGTH	32 mg.
ANACIN-3 TABLETS	32 mg.
BIO SLIM T CAPSULES	140 mg.
CENEGESIC	15 mg.
COPE	32 mg.
CORYBAN-D	30 mg.
DEX-A-DIET II	200 mg.
DEXATRIM	200 mg.
DEXATRIM EXTRA STRENGTH	200 mg.
DIETAC CAPSULES	200 mg.
DRISTAN A-F DECONGESTANT TABLETS	16.2 mg.
DRISTAN DECONGESTANT TABLETS	16.2 mg.
DURADYNE-FORTE	30 mg.
EUPHENEX	15 mg.
EXCEDRIN	64.8 mg.
GOODY'S HEADACHE POWDER	32.5 mg.
HERBAL DIURETIC TABLETS	16.2 mg.
HISTA-COMPOUND NO. 5	32.5 mg.
HUNGREX PLUS	66 mg.
MIDOL	32.4 mg.
MIDRAN DECONGESTANT	32.5 mg.
NEO-SYNEPHRINE COMPOUND	15 mg.
NODOZ	100 mg.
PROLAMINE	140 mg.
SINAPILS	32.4 mg.
SLIM ONE CAPSULES	200 mg.

STANBACK ANALGESIC POWDERS	15 mg.
SUPER-DECON	32 mg.
TRIAMINICIN	30 mg.
VANQUISH	33 mg.
VIVARIN	200 mg.

FOR A QUICK COMPARISON

COFFEE	*PER CUP*
Instant	66 mg.
Percolated	110 mg.
Drip	155 mg.

TEA

Black 1-minute brew	28 mg.
Black 5-minute brew	46 mg.

SOFT DRINKS	*12-OUNCE CAN OR BOTTLE*
Coca-Cola	64.7 mg.
Dr. Pepper	60.9 mg.
Mountain Dew	54.7 mg.
Diet Dr. Pepper	54.2 mg.
Tab	49.4 mg.
Pepsi-Cola	43.1 mg.
R.C. Cola	33.7 mg.
Diet R.C.	33.0 mg.
Diet-Rite	31.7 mg.

CHOCOLATE	*1 OUNCE*
Milk chocolate	6 mg.
Baking chocolate	25 mg.
Cocoa (1 cup)	5–10 mg.

REMEMBER: Caffeine is a drug (one quart of coffee consumed in three hours can destroy much of the body's thiamin, vitamin B_1), and it *can be toxic*. Ten grams can be lethal!

23. And don't forget hidden sugars and saccharin

In most drugs the sugar and/or saccharin content is relatively unimportant, because few products are taken in large doses over a long period of time—but antacids are an exception. They're usually ingested on a fairly regular basis. So, if you think you've had upset stomachs before, just wait until you look at this unsettling list!

PRODUCT	SUGAR PER TABLESPOON	SACCHARIN PER TABLESPOON
ALTERNAGEL LIQUID	2,000 mg.	–
ALUDROX LIQUID	150 mg.	5.25 mg.
ALUDROX TABLETS	368 mg.	1.9 mg.
AMPHOJEL LIQUID	60 mg.	–
AMPHOJEL TABLETS, 0.3 g	24 mg.	0.155 mg.
AMPHOJEL TABLETS, 0.6 g	48 mg.	0.31 mg.
BASALJEL LIQUID	–	1.5 mg.
BASALJEL CAPSULES OR TABLETS	41 mg.	–
BASALJEL EXTRA STRENGTH LIQUID	375 mg.	7.5 mg.
CAMALOX LIQUID	–	2.25 mg.
CAMALOX TABLETS	–	1.5 mg.
GAVISCON LIQUID	1,500 mg.	2.4 mg.
GAVISCON TABLETS	1,200 mg.	–
GAVISCON-2 TABLETS	2,400 mg.	–
GELUSIL LIQUID	–	2.25 mg.
GELUSIL TABLETS	280 mg.	–
GELUSIL M TABLETS	265 mg.	–
GELUSIL II TABLETS	116 mg.	1.0 mg.
MAALOX LIQUID	–	4.2 mg.
MAALOX NO. 1 TABLETS	–	1.0 mg.
MAALOX NO. 2 TABLETS	145 mg.	3.0 mg.
MAALOX PLUS LIQUID	–	3.3 mg.
MAALOX PLUS TABLETS	575 mg.	1.5 mg.
MAALOX THERAPEUTIC CONCENTRATE LIQUID	–	–
MYLANTA LIQUID	2,000 mg.	

MYLANTA TABLETS	275 mg.	–
MYLANTA-II LIQUID	2,000 mg.	–
MYLANTA-II TABLETS	918 mg.	1.5 mg.
OXAINE LIQUID	150 mg.	1.5 mg.
PHILLIPS' MILK OF MAGNESIA, FLAVORED	–	5.78 mg.
PHILLIPS' MILK OF MAGNESIA TABLETS	195 mg.	–
PHOSPHALJEL LIQUID	–	–
RIOPAN LIQUID	–	4.05 mg.
RIOPAN CHEW TABLETS	70 mg.	–
RIOPAN SWALLOW TABLETS	–	0.1 mg.
RIOPAN PLUS LIQUID	–	4.05 mg.
RIOPAN PLUS CHEW TABLETS	610 mg.	–
SILAIN-GEL LIQUID	–	0.75 mg.
SIMECO LIQUID	129 mg.	–
TRISOGEL TABLETS	–	–

FOR A QUICK COMPARISON

APPROXIMATE TEASPOONS OF SUGAR PER SERVING
(3 TEASPOONS = 1 TABLESPOON)

DRINKS	12-OUNCE CAN OR BOTTLE
Coca-Cola	7 tsp.
Ginger ale	10 tsp.
Seven-Up	7½ tsp.
Sweet cider	9 tsp.

CAKES	4 OUNCES
Angel food	7 tsp.
Applesauce cake	5½ tsp.
Cheesecake	2 tsp.
Chocolate cake (iced)	10 tsp.
Coffee cake	4 tsp.
Pound cake	5 tsp.
Sponge cake	8 tsp.

COOKIES	1 WHOLE
Fig Newtons	5 tsp.
Gingersnaps	3 tsp.
Macaroons	6 tsp.
Chocolate eclair	7 tsp.
Doughnut (glazed)	6 tsp.

24. The lowdown on drug allergies

All allergies are hypersensitivities to specific substances that, in the same or similar amounts, do not bother other people. The substance which causes the allergy is known as an antigen or an allergen. In an allergic situation, your inner defense mechanisms produce *antibodies* to fight off the invading antigens; but when the antigens are drugs designed to help you, your system's antibodies (ordinarily the good guys) become hazardous to your health.

Drug allergies are widespread and on the increase, as medicines become more and more complex. And most people are allergic not just to one brand-name product, but to a whole chemical class of drugs. (If you're allergic to *penicillin*, you'll probably be allergic to *empicillin*, too. The same holds true for other drug classes, such as barbiturates, cortisone drugs, etc.)

> Just because you've had no adverse reaction to a medication in the past doesn't mean that you can't develop a hypersensitivity to it in the future.

Allergic reactions to medicines are as varied as the medicines themselves, but the most common effects are:

- dermatitis (especially in the case of topical medications that are applied directly to the skin)
- itching
- rashes
- asthma (contraction of smooth muscles in the small tubes of the lungs)

The most extreme allergic reaction to a drug is anaphylactic shock, which can be fatal if not treated quickly (usually by injection of *epinephrine*). Symptoms include extreme difficulty in breathing, severe itching, coughing, increased pulse rate, and a bluish tinge to the skin, which may be followed by convulsions or unconsciousness.

25. Drug allergy facts you should know

- Drug reactions can occur suddenly (within minutes), or may appear slowly, sometimes several weeks after you've been on a medication.
- The kind of allergic reaction you get doesn't necessarily depend on how the medication was given. (A drug taken orally might cause asthma, while an injection of an antibiotic might merely result in hives.)
- Generally, allergic responses are more severe if a substance is injected.
- Mild allergic reactions to a medication you've taken in the past should be brought to your doctor's attention before you take the drug again to avoid a more serious allergic reaction, such as anaphylactic shock.
- Even if you have no personal or family history of any kind of allergy, you can still develop a hypersensitivity to a drug.
- Any unusual reaction to your medication should be brought to your doctor's attention immediately.
- If you have an allergy to any antibiotic pills, beware of ointments containing that same antibiotic.
- One of the most common drug allergies is to one of the most widely used medications—*aspirin*.
- If you're allergic to *aspirin*, be aware that it's an ingredient in hundreds of medicines, OTC and prescription, so be sure to check out every medication you take with your pharmacist, doctor, or a drug guide that lists all ingredients (see sections 32–52).
- Along with *aspirin*, other drugs that most often prompt allergic reaction are *penicillin*, sulfonamides, *streptomycin*, and barbiturates.

26. Foods and supplements that can help alleviate drug allergies

The following food and supplement regimen might not eliminate a drug allergy, but it can aid in preventing hypersensitivities and help reduce uncomfortable drug reactions.

INCREASE THESE FOODS IN YOUR DIET

Citrus fruits and juices, nutritional yeast, liver, fish liver oil, soy products, and alfalfa sprouts

SUPPLEMENTS ·

High-potency multiple vitamin with chelated minerals (time-release preferable)	2 times daily
Vitamin C	1,000 mg. 2 times daily
Vitamin B-complex	100 mg. 3 times daily
Pantothenic acid	1,000 mg. 2 times daily

27. Drugs and your lifestyle

Before you start on any drug regimen, it's important to consider how that particular drug (its dosage, the times of day you take it) is going to interact with your lifestyle.

Be sure you know how you're going to react to a medication, by taking it first in a safe at home situation, so that you can weigh its advantages and disadvantages. Various pain-killers, for instance, might cause you to become drowsy and fuzzy-headed, dangerous reactions if you're a truck driver or someone who operates machinery. So if you intend to take medicine and want to carry on with your life in a normal, safe fashion, discuss the drug in this light with your doctor or pharmacist.

- Find out if there is an alternative medication with side effects less likely to interfere with the way you live.
- Ask if the medication can be taken on a different schedule and still be effective.
- Know how long a particular drug will be active in your

system and discuss the possibility of missing a dose in order to effectively perform some daily task.

• Consult with a nutritionally-oriented doctor (see section 167) to find out if there is some natural remedy for your condition that won't interfere with your job or your life. (See "Nature's Pharmacy" in sections 32–52.)

28. Any questions about Chapter IV?

When a doctor asks me if I'm allergic to the drug he's prescribing, how am I supposed to know if I've never taken the drug before? I broke out in a terrible rash after taking penicillin for the first time. Couldn't this have been avoided by some sort of test?

Unfortunately, there is still no *sure* way of knowing whether or not a patient will have an allergic reaction to a drug. Most doctors have to rely heavily on your medical history and potential for allergic reactions in general. But there is a skin test for sensitivity to *penicillin* that's fairly reliable. (Skin tests for other drugs haven't been successful, because the exact derivative or breakdown product of the drug isn't known.) The test is called Pre-Pen, but right now it's being used only on a very limited basis. The National Institute of Allergy and Infectious Diseases feels confident, though, that it will be widely available within the next few years.

I'm a diabetic, and whenever I give myself an insulin shot I break out in a mild case of hives. Is this a common reaction?

It's a common *allergic* reaction. In some cases, it's due to the pork or beef protein from which the hormone is derived; in others, it's due to components such as zinc, which is often used in commercial *insulin*. Ask your doctor about zinc-free *insulin*, which is now available. Also inquire about HUMULIN, which consists of a true human *insulin* derived from DNA technology. This new *insulin* product is now available and is expected to cause a much lower incidence of drug allergies.

Is it true that you can have an allergic reaction to drugs that make your hair fall out?

Yes. And some drugs more than others seem to elicit this

sort of dermatologic allergy. The ones most likely to do so are: HALDOL (*haloperidol*), a tranquilizer; ZYLOPRIM (*allopurinol*), an antigout drug; COUMADIN (*warfarin sodium*), an anticoagulant; INDERAL (*propranolol*), a beta-blocking agent used to treat high blood pressure and certain heart conditions; and DEPAKENE (*valproic acid*), an antiepileptic drug.

Part Two

ABECEDARY OF PILLS AND POTIONS

Chapter V

Any Body's Guide to Medications

29. What kind of drug is this anyway?

Millions of people take thousands of drugs every year and are still confused about what *type* of drugs they're taking. They'll refer to their medications as "heart pills," or "water pills," or "pain pills," for instance, and be totally at a loss when asked if they've been taking an antianginal or an analgesic, an antacid or an antihistamine. But because these are the type of classifications that drugs fall under, it's important to know the difference between them.

The following is a list of drug categories, alphabetized and explained for quick reference:

AMEBICIDES—specific antibiotics to fight internal parasites, such as those that cause malaria and other sorts of extra-intestinal illnesses. (Trichomonacides are also amebicides, but specifically for treatment of monilial and trichomonal vaginal infections.)

ANALEPTIC AGENTS—central nervous stimulants used mostly to enhance the mental and physical activity of elderly patients.

ANALGESICS—any drugs used to relieve pain.

ANESTHETICS—drugs used to prevent the conduction of nerve impulses (when injected) to deaden pain. (General anesthetics can bring on unconsciousness to eliminate pain.) Anesthetics can also be applied topically or inserted rectally to numb afflicted areas.

ANOREXICS or APPETITE SUPPRESSANTS—central nervous system stimulants, such as amphetamines, used in the treatment of obesity; "diet pills."

ANTACIDS—drugs used to neutralize acids, primarily those involved in digestion.

ANTHELMINTICS—drugs used to rid the body of worms (pinworms, roundworms, whipworms, hookworms, etc.)

ANTIALCOHOL PREPARATIONS—drugs that produce a highly unpleasant reaction when the patient ingests even small amounts of alcohol. Used in the treatment of alcoholism.

ANTIANGINALS—cardiovascular drugs used specifically to alleviate and prevent chest pain due to angina attacks.

ANTIARRHYTHMICS—also cardiovascular drugs, but used primarily to regulate arrhythmic heart conditions.

ANTIARTHRITICS—drugs used to combat the pain and inflammation of joints in arthritis.

ANTIASTHMA DRUGS—drugs used to relax the smooth muscle of the bronchial airways and pulmonary blood vessels to facilitate breathing in asthmatic patients.

ANTIBACTERIALS—drugs used in the treatment of specific bacterial infections, those not responsive to ordinary antibiotics.

ANTIBIOTICS—the general group of drugs, usually prepared from molds or moldlike organisms, which are used in the treatment of infections.

ANTICOAGULANTS—drugs which reduce the clotting tendencies of the blood.

ANTICONVULSANTS—drugs used for the control and prevention of convulsions and seizures.

ANTIDEPRESSANTS—mood-elevating medications.

ANTIDIABETICS—drugs used in the treatment of diabetes.

ANTIDIARRHEALS—preparations to treat severe diarrhea.

ANTIDYSKINETICS—drugs used in the treatment of Parkinson's disease.

ANTIFLATULENTS—drugs used to diminish intestinal gas.

ANTIFUNGALS—drugs used to combat fungus infections.

ANTIHISTAMINES—drugs used to treat symptoms of allergies (such as runny nose, watery eyes, etc.).

ANTIHYPERLIPIDEMICS—drugs used to reduce high blood cholesterol levels.

ANTIHYPERTENSIVES—drugs used to lower blood pressure.

ANTI-INFLAMMATORIES—drugs used to counteract or diminish inflammation, especially in arthritis.

ANTINAUSEANTS—drugs used to prevent nausea and motion sickness.

ANTINEOPLASTICS—drugs used to prevent the growth and development of malignant (cancerous) cells.

ANTIPARASITICS—medications to treat scabies and lice infections, as well as internal parasites.

ANTIPRURITICS—medications to help relieve itching.

ANTIPSYCHOTICS—drugs used to treat nervous, mental, and emotional conditions.

ANTIPYRETICS—drugs used to lower fever.

ANTISPASMODICS or ANTICHOLINERGICS—drugs used to relieve cramping and spasms of the stomach, intestines, and bladder.

ANTITUSSIVES—drugs used to relieve coughs.

ANTI-URIC ACIDS—drugs which reduce high levels of uric acid in blood and treat gout.

BIOLOGICALS—substances of organic origin which include vaccines, immunization serums, and allergenic extracts used for diagnosis and therapy in allergies.

BRONCHIAL DILATORS—drugs used in the treatment of bronchial asthma, bronchitis, and emphysema to relieve wheezing and shortness of breath.

CARDIOVASCULAR PREPARATIONS—medications used to treat heart problems. Antianginals, Antiarrhythmics, Beta and Calcium Blockers, and Vasodilators are in this category.

CONTRACEPTIVES (oral)—these are estrogens and progestins, hormones that change the body's hormone balance, which prevents pregnancy.

DECONGESTANTS and EXPECTORANTS—cough and cold preparations to relieve sinus and bronchial congestion.

DERMATOLOGICALS—topical medications for the treatment of acne and other infections of the skin.

DIURETICS—drugs which reduce the amount of water in the body by increasing the flow of urine. Commonly used in the treatment of high blood pressure, kidney malfunction, and congestive heart failure, among other conditions.

ELECTROLYTES—substances such as sodium, potassium, and chlorides that are normally found in the blood. Supplements of any of these, most commonly potassium, are usually prescribed for patients who've lost too much through poor diet, illness, or medication.

EMETICS—taken to cause vomiting, an emergency treatment for certain kinds of poisoning.

ESTROGENS—female hormones used as menstrual cycle regulators, contraceptives (usually when in conjunction with progestins), in the treatment of menopausal symptoms and certain types of breast and prostate cancer.

GERIATRICS—drugs used to treat symptoms of mental decline in older persons.

GERMICIDES—preparations that destroy germs.

HEMATINICS—therapeutic medications for the blood.

HEMOSTATICS—drugs used to treat excessive bleeding that is caused by certain conditions.

HORMONES—chemicals that originate in the glands and are transported by the blood to all parts of the body. Hormones such as *estrogen* are used in the treatment of menstrual irregularity and for alleviating menopausal discomfort; *estrogen* and *progestogen* combinations are used in birth control pills.

HYPNOTICS—essentially sleeping pills, used in the treatment of insomnia.

LAXATIVES—drugs used to relieve constipation by facilitating bowel movements.

MUCOLYTICS—drugs used to decongest swollen mucous membranes when there is severe congestion.

MUSCLE RELAXANTS—drugs used primarily to relieve spasms, tightness and cramping of muscles caused by disease or injury.

OPHTHALMOLOGICALS—medications for the eyes.

OTIC PREPARATIONS—medicines for the ears.

OXYTOCICS—synthetic hormones used to stimulate the contraction of the uterus.

PEDICULICIDES—like antiparasitics these medicines are used to kill head, body, and pubic (crab) lice.

PSYCHOSTIMULANTS—drugs used in the treatment of narcolepsy, and behavior problems in hyperactive children.

SEDATIVES—calming agents, used to decrease anxiety; in sufficient doses they will act as hypnotics.

SULFONAMIDES—a group of sulfa drugs used to treat specific infections that are not responsive to other antibacterials.

SYMPATHOMIMETICS—drugs used to raise blood pressure, relieve congestion; produces stimulation akin to that of the sympathetic nervous system.

THYROID PREPARATIONS—drugs used for treatment of underactive and overactive thyroid conditions.

TRANQUILIZERS—sedatives that decrease anxiety (or other psychic disturbances) without sedating to the point of sleep.

URICOSURIC AGENTS—drugs used to treat chronic gout and other medical problems that cause too much uric acid to be produced by the body.

30. Are you in the top 200—and do you know why?

Like records and books, drugs have their best-seller list too. But when you look over the pharmaceutical popularity poll that follows and realize how many medicines are being prescribed for anxiety, high blood pressure, heart disease, and stomach disorders, it makes you wonder what we're doing wrong. Personally, I think it's filling and refilling those prescriptions without even inquiring about alternatives.

As a pharmacist and a nutritionist, I'm appalled at the increasing number of Rxs being written for drugs, when in many instances prescriptions for dietary changes would serve the same—if not a better—purpose. At the very least, specific natural foods should be prescribed along with drugs to minimize side effects and maximize effectiveness, keeping treatments with potentially harmful chemicals as short as possible. (See sections 32–52.)

Take a look at 1982's top 200 and see if any of your medications are on it; then check the lowdown on those drugs in the section indicated on the right. Chances are there's a lot more you should know than you do about those popular pills you're popping.

THE 200 BESTSELLING DRUGS
IN ALPHABETICAL ORDER

Product Name	See Section . . .
ACHROMYCIN V	33
ACTIFED	38
ACTIFED-C EXPECTORANT	47
ALDACTAZIDE	40
ALDACTONE	40
ALDOMET	40
ALDORIL	40
AMBENYL EXPECTORANT	47
AMCILL	33
Aminophylline	52
Amitriptyline HCl	35
Amoxicillin	33
AMOXIL	33
AMPICILLIN	33
ANTIVERT	42
ANUSOL-HC	52
APRESOLINE	40
ARTANE	52
ATARAX	38, 42
ATIVAN	50
ATROMID-S	39
BACTRIM	33
BACTRIM DS	33
BENADRYL CAPS/TABS	38
BENADRYL ELIXIR	38
BENDECTIN	42
BENTYL	43

TUSS-ORNADE	47
TYLENOL/CODEINE	32
VALISONE	52
VALIUM	50
VANCERIL	41
VASODILAN	46
V-CILLIN K	33
VIBRAMYCIN	33
VIBRA-TABS	33
VISTARIL	50
ZAROXOLYN	40
ZYLOPRIM	44

31. Any questions about Chapter V?

What are the most popularly prescribed drugs?

According to a tabulation made by Pharmaceutical Data Service, the top 10 drugs prescribed in the United States (as of 1983) are as follows:

1. INDERAL
2. LANOXIN
3. DYAZIDE
4. VALIUM
5. TYLENOL w/ CODEINE
6. LASIX
7. TAGAMET
8. MOTRIN
9. ORTHO-NOVUM
10. KEFLEX

If a drug is listed among the top 10 most prescribed medications, would you say that it's safer than a similar drug that's prescribed less often?

Not necessarily. All drugs that are on the market have had to meet equivalent FDA standards—and *no* drugs are risk free. In fact, TAGAMET, which is one of the top 10 most prescribed drugs in the United States, has recently come into question as to whether it can safely be prescribed for pregnant women. Researchers in Pittsburgh have found that the male offspring of rats given *cimetidine* (TAGAMET) during pregnancy showed decreased weight of their sexual organs at puberty and disturbed sexual patterns. There's still a controversy on the role of sex steroid imprinting on the human fetal brain, but it's advised that the drug be used with caution by pregnant women.

More often than not, it isn't a drug's effectiveness or safety that puts it into the top ten, but the drug company's effective promotion and persuasive salespeople.

Chapter VI

Medicines From A to Z

NOTE: The drugs mentioned in this chapter are among those most commonly prescribed in the United States. If your particular medication is not listed, check the index for a possible cross-reference to its category, or consult one of the guides listed in the bibliography for further information. Also, keep in mind that the foods and supplements recommended are not prescriptive nor intended as medical advice.

32. Analgesics (pain relievers)

WHAT THEY DO

- Relieve pain and can also reduce fever, since most contain either *aspirin* or *acetaminophen*.
- Analgesics containing *aspirin* will also work against inflammation, which *acetaminophen* will not.

WHAT THEY'RE USED FOR

- Injuries
- Backaches

- Arthritis
- Postoperative relief
- Headaches
- Menstrual cramps
- Toothaches

POSSIBLE SIDE EFFECTS

Dizziness, nausea, indigestion, drowsiness, loss of appetite, insomnia, skin rash, nervousness, dry mouth, constipation, blurred vision, diarrhea. (For foods and vitamins that can help combat side effects, see section 54.)

SOME BRAND NAMES	GENERIC NAME	SPECIAL NOTES
DARVOCET-N	*propoxyphene napsylate & acetaminophen*	can be *extremely* dangerous if taken with alcohol, sedatives, tranquilizers or any nervous system depressants
DARVON	*Propoxyphene hydrochloride*	same as above
DARVON COMPOUND	*Propoxyphene hydrochloride & APC (the* abbreviation for *aspirin, phenacetin,* and *caffeine)*	same as above
DOLOBID	*Diflunisal*	
EMPIRIN	*Aspirin* 325 mg. (5 grs.)	
EMPIRIN w/ *codeine*	*Aspirin & codeine*	may cause unusual excitement in children

SOME BRAND NAMES	GENERIC NAME	SPECIAL NOTES
EQUAGESIC	Meprobamate, ethoheptazine, & aspirin	
FIORINAL	Butalbital & APC	may cause clumsiness
FIORINAL w/ codeine	Butalbital, APC, & codeine	may cause clumsiness
NORGESIC FORTE	Orphenadrine & APC	may cause drowsiness; can cause diabetics to obtain false test results with urine sugar tests; will increase the effects of alcohol and any medicines that slow down the nervous system
PERCOCET-5	Oxycodone hydrochloride & acetaminophen	
PERCODAN	Oxycodone & aspirin	
PERCODAN-DEMI	Oxycodone & aspirin	
PHENAPHEN w/codeine	Acetaminophen & codeine	
PYRIDIUM	Phenazopyridine hydrochloride	relieves pain of urinary tract infections, but does not cure infection; may cause false test results on urine sugar analyses; can change color of urine

SOME BRAND NAMES	GENERIC NAME	SPECIAL NOTES
SYNALGOS-DC	*Drocode, promethazine, & APC*	may cause painful urination
TALWIN	*Pentazocine*	may cause hallucinations & mental confusion; extended use can lead to drug dependency
TYLENOL w/ codeine	*Acetaminophen & codeine*	
VICODIN	*Hydrocodone bitartrate & acetaminophen*	may cause mood changes, fear, & psychological dependence

FOODS THAT CAN INCREASE EFFECTIVENESS

whole wheat, peanuts, liver, eggs, milk, cantaloupe, beef, pork, citrus fruits, green & leafy vegetables (contain vitamins and minerals that can act as natural analgesics)

FOODS THAT CAN DECREASE EFFECTIVENESS

brussels sprouts, cabbage, charcoal broiled foods (can interfere with effectiveness of acetaminophen and phenacetin); carbohydrates such as crackers, jellies, candies, etc. (can slow medicine's absorption rate)

CAUTIONS

- Consult your doctor before taking any analgesic if you are currently taking any antihistamines (or cold or allergy medications), sedatives, tranquilizers, barbiturates, seizure medicines, other pain medicines, or tricyclic antidepressants, especially if you have taken any MAO drugs (monoamine-oxidase inhibitors) within the previous two weeks.

- Do not take an analgesic if you're pregnant, think you're pregnant, or a nursing mother, without consulting your doctor about the risks involved.
- Most analgesics contain at least one or more of the following ingredients: *aspirin, acetaminophen, phenacetin,* and *caffeine.* Check your prescription's ingredients (ask your doctor, pharmacist, or consult a reputable drug reference work) to make sure you're not allergic to any of them.
- **Long-term use of *any* prescription analgesic can cause serious drug tolerance and/or dependence (see sections 85, 86).**
- Some analgesics, such as SYNALGOS-DC and drugs with *codeine,* are respiratory depressants, and should be used with extreme caution by anyone who has breathing difficulties.
- The *aspirin* content of an analgesic can adversely affect anticoagulant medications (blood thinners) by increasing the effectiveness of the anticoagulant, enough to cause severe bleeding.
- Any narcotic analgesic (e.g., VICODIN, PERCODAN, PERCOCET-5) should not be taken for abdominal pain, or in the case of pain due to head injury, without first consulting a doctor, since the respiratory depressant effects of narcotics may produce adverse reactions and also obscure proper medical diagnosis of the condition.
- Narcotic analgesics should be used cautiously by elderly patients and anyone with liver and kidney problems.
- **Do not drink alcohol while taking pain-killers! Certain combinations (e.g. alcohol with propoxyphene) can be deadly even in small doses.**

NATURE'S PHARMACY

- Vitamin B_1 (thiamine) can help relieve dental postoperative pain.
- Biotin helps ease muscle pains.
- Vitamin C aids in healing wounds, burns, and bleeding gums.
- Pantothenic acid (1,000 mg. daily) can reduce arthritis pain.

- Folic acid can act as a natural analgesic.
- Niacin can help prevent and ease severity of migraine headaches.
- PABA (para-aminobenzoic acid) can reduce the pain of burns.
- L-tryptophan has been found to have pain-relieving properties.
- Phosphorus can lessen pain caused by arthritis.

(For a quick reference list of foods that contain the vitamins and minerals mentioned, see section 55.)

MY ADVICE

- Analgesics that contain *aspirin* will cause less digestive upset if taken when there's food in the stomach—or when taken with a *full* glass of water.
- When taking analgesics containing *aspirin*, avoid combining them with acidic foods, such as citrus fruits and juices and alcoholic drinks, which can increase the irritating effects on the stomach and cause gastric bleeding.
- Most analgesics cause drowsiness and can take effect within a half-hour (and can last between 4 and 6 hours), so don't take a pill and plan on driving anywhere unless you know for sure how you respond to the medication.

33. Antibiotics

WHAT THEY DO

- Kill or effectively inhibit the growth of bacteria and various other microorganisms (including some fungi).

WHAT THEY'RE USED FOR

- Infections (systemic & topical)
- Preventives before and after surgery
- Protective therapy for individuals with congenital heart disease, rheumatic heart disease, or other conditions where the possibility of infection can be extremely dangerous

- As preventives to ward off secondary infections during viral illnesses, against which (with a few exceptions) antibiotics are *not* effective. (They do *not* work on colds or flu.)

POSSIBLE SIDE EFFECTS

Nausea, diarrhea, vomiting (less common with *amoxicillin, cloxacillin, dicloxacillin, methicillin, nafcillin,* and *oxacillin*), rectal or genital itching, vaginal discharge, stomach cramps, brown or black discoloration of tongue and sensitivity to sunlight (particularly with *tetracyclines*), excessive thirst, increased urination, decreased urination, hives, and bruising of skin. (For foods and vitamins that can help combat side effects, see section 54.)

SOME BRAND NAMES	GENERIC NAME	SPECIAL NOTES
ACHROMYCIN V	Tetracycline	
AMCILL	Ampicillin	
AMOXIL SUSP.	Amoxicillin	
BACTRIM-DS	Trimethoprim & sulfamethoxazole	
CECLOR	Cefaclor	
CINOBAC	Cinoxacin	
CLAFORAN	Cefotaxime sodium	
CORTISPORIN OTIC	Hydrocortisone, neomycin sulfate, polymyxin-B	contains a steroid to reduce inflammation
E.E.S.	Erythromycin	
E-MYCIN	Erythromycin	
ERYPAR	Erythromycin	
ERYTHROCIN	Erythromycin	
ERYTHROMYCIN BASE FILMTAB	Erythromycin	

SOME BRAND NAMES	GENERIC NAME	SPECIAL NOTES
ETHRIL	Erythromycin	
FLAGYL	Metronidazole	increases the effect of anticoagulants; may darken urine & cause incontinence; do not drink alcohol while on medicine
GANTRISIN	Sulfisoxazole	drinking extra water helps prevent unwanted side effects
GYNE-LOTRIMIN	Clotrimazole	an antifungal vaginal medication; if response to treatment is poor, lab tests should be repeated to confirm original diagnosis
ILOSONE	Erythromycin estolate	
KEFLEX	Cephalexin	should be taken cautiously by anyone sensitive to drugs in general & to penicillin in particular
LAROTID	Amoxicillin	
LEDERCILLIN VK	Penicillin V potassium	
LOTRIMIN CREAM	Clotrimazole	topical, broad-spectrum antifungal

SOME BRAND NAMES	GENERIC NAME	SPECIAL NOTES
MACRODANTIN	Nitrofurantoin macrocrystals	
MEZLIN	Mezlocillin sodium	
MONISTAT CREAM	Miconazole nitrate	a regimen of 7 or more days has a cure rate equivalent to former 14-day regimens
MOXAM	Moxalactam disodium	
NIZORAL	Ketoconazole	
OMNIPEN	Ampicillin	
PEN-VEE K	Penicillin V potassium	
SEPTRA-DS	Trimethoprim, sulfamethoxazole	
SK-AMPICILLIN	Ampicillin	
SK PENICILLIN VK	Penicillin V potassium	
SK TETRA-CYCLINE	Tetracycline	
SPECTROBID	Bacampicillin	
SUMYCIN	Tetracycline	
TETRACYCLINE CAPS	Tetracycline	
V-CILLIN K	Penicillin V potassium	
VIBRAMYCIN	Doxycycline	
VIBRA-TABS	Doxycycline	

FOODS THAT CAN INCREASE EFFECTIVENESS

fish, liver, eggs, green leafy vegetables, milk, whole grains, citrus fruits. (Not effective for anyone taking *griseofulvin*, which is least well absorbed on a high protein diet.) (NOTE: These are foods to include in diet, not to take *with* medicines. Most antibiotics should be taken on an empty stomach without fruit juices or milk. (See section 19.) For exceptions see CAUTIONS.)

FOODS THAT CAN DECREASE EFFECTIVENESS

milk, dairy products, and sardines decrease the effectiveness of *tetracyclines* (except for VIBRAMYCIN, which is *doxycycline*). Citrus fruits and juices, pickles, tomatoes, colas, wine, and caffeine can decrease the effectiveness of *erythromycin, penicillin*, and *ampicillin*, if the foods and medicines are taken together.

CAUTIONS

- Do not take any antibiotic if you have a history of hypersensitivity to *penicillin,* any other drugs, or allergies in general, without consulting your doctor.
- If you're pregnant, trying to become pregnant, or a nursing mother, consult your doctor before taking any antibiotic.
- Take medicine for full time of treatment, *even if symptoms disappear!* (A "strep" infection usually takes 10 to 14 days.)
- Don't overuse an antibiotic, or you run the risk of allowing more resistant strains to develop in the future.
- One antibiotic is not interchangeable with another, so make sure you've checked with your doctor on which one is right for your present infection.
- Antibiotics should be taken on an *empty* stomach, which means at least one hour before or two hours after meals. (Some exceptions are VIBRAMYCIN and antifungals such as FULVICIN and GRISACTIN, which should be taken *with* meals.)

- Do not take *tetracyclines* (except for *doxycycline*) with milk or dairy products.
- Do not take *penicillin, ampicillin, cloxacillin,* or *erythromycin* with fruit juice.
- Stay out of the sun if you're taking *tetracycline*, because you run the risk of sunburn even from a short exposure.

NATURE'S PHARMACY

- Garlic, vitamin C, and (don't laugh, it's true) chicken soup have remarkable natural antibiotic properties.
- Vitamin A can build resistance to respiratory infections.
- Pantothenic acid can fight infections by building antibodies and also reduce the adverse effects of many antibiotics.
- Folic acid can help protect you against intestinal parasites and food poisoning.

(For a quick reference list of foods that contain the vitamins and minerals mentioned, see section 55.)

MY ADVICE

- If you're taking *tetracycline*, PABA (para-aminobenzoic acid) ointment is high among those that are most effective for preventing sunburn.
- Antibiotics don't always kill just the bad bacteria, and often kill off friendly intestinal bacteria, causing diarrhea and an overgrowth of the fungus monilia abricans. This fungus can grow in the intestines, vagina, lungs, mouth (thrush), on the fingers, or under the nails. A few days use of generous amounts of acidophilus culture, though, can clear this up.
- Attention, travelers! If you've suffered from Montezuma's Revenge (traveler's diarrhea) and have been disappointed in the often-prescribed treatment of VIBRAMYCIN and Pepto-Bismol, you should know that when *doxycycline* is taken with Pepto-Bismol, the effectiveness of the antibiotic is substantially reduced—even when the Pepto-Bismol is taken two hours before. The trick, which your doctor

might have forgotten to mention, is to take the Pepto-Bismol two hours *after* taking the antibiotic!

- Let me stress this: If you don't *need* an antibiotic, don't take it! You're getting more than you think already. Doctors have found that the large doses of antibiotics fed to cattle, hogs, and chickens have produced three new strains of very hearty bacteria which eventually come through to us, and which are highly resistant to or unaffected by antibiotics!

- Parents, don't pressure your pediatrician for a prescription for antibiotics over the phone. According to an intensive study of 4,700 infants in Canada, upper respiratory infections, when they occur in children under three, are rarely bacterial in nature. (Remember that antibiotics are not effective against viral infections, which colds and flu are!) It's extremely unlikely that a sore throat is an emergency, so delaying antibiotic treatment for 12 to 24 hours (time to identify the bacteria) is well worth the wait.

- None of the *tetracycline* antibiotics (those with generic names ending in *line*) should be given to children under the age of 8 or taken by pregnant or nursing mothers since these drugs can cause tooth discoloration in children.

34. Anticoagulants (blood thinners)

WHAT THEY DO

- Decrease the clotting ability of the blood.
- Help prevent potentially harmful clots from forming in blood vessels.

WHAT THEY'RE USED FOR

- Severe thrombophlebitis
- Lung diseases
- Heart diseases
- Various blood-vessel conditions

POSSIBLE SIDE EFFECTS

Bloated stomach, stomach cramps, loss of appetite, backaches, dizziness, black tarry stools, cloudy or bloody urine, constipation, continuing headaches, dark-colored vomit (almost any of these side effects could indicate internal bleeding, so notify your doctor immediately), loss of hair, nausea, skin rash, itching, a syndrome called "purple toes," hives, continued erection without sexual desire. (For foods and vitamins that can help combat side effects, see section 54.)

SOME BRAND NAMES	GENERIC NAME	SPECIAL NOTES
COUMADIN	*Warfarin sodium*	
PANWARFIN	*Warfarin sodium*	
PANHEPRIN	*Heparin sodium*	supplied by injection

FOODS THAT CAN INCREASE EFFECTIVENESS	FOODS THAT CAN DECREASE EFFECTIVENESS
citrus fruits and juices, chicken, cottage cheese, skim milk (contain vitamins that lower incidence of blood clots)	kelp, alfalfa, egg yolk, safflower oil, fish liver oils, spinach, dark green leafy vegetables (high in vitamin K and can reverse anticoagulant effectiveness)

CAUTIONS

- Consult your doctor before taking an anticoagulant if you have any other medical problems; your physical state can influence your response to the drug.
- Don't take an anticoagulant if you are pregnant, trying to become pregnant, or are a nursing mother.
- Before beginning anticoagulant therapy, be sure to let your doctor know if you've recently made any changes in your diet, incurred any injuries, had a fever, diarrhea, heavy menstrual bleeding, X-ray treatment, medical or dental surgery, or the insertion of an IUD (intrauterine device).

- Don't take *any* OTC or other medications without first checking with your pharmacist or doctor! (*Aspirin,* antacids, and laxatives, in particular, can seriously affect the way anticoagulant medications work and cause dangerous— even life threatening—situations.)
- Dosages of anticoagulants are highly individualized, and patients undergoing therapy *must not* ignore appointments for laboratory monitoring of prothrombin (clotting) time.
- Be aware that COUMADIN and PANWARFIN (*warfarin sodium*) are potent drugs with a half-life (the time it remains in the body) of two-and-a-half days, which means that their effects can become more pronounced as daily doses overlap.

NATURE'S PHARMACY

- Vitamin C can lower incidence of blood clots in veins.
- Vitamin E aids in preventing and dissolving blood clots.

(For a quick reference list of foods that contain the vitamins and minerals mentioned, see section 55.)

MY ADVICE

- Though vitamin C can lower the incidence of blood clots in veins, I don't advise it as a supplement during anticoagulant therapy without consulting your doctor. It can cause a change in clotting time and throw off results of laboratory tests.
- Make sure you understand your doctor's instructions on taking the drug and keep him or her informed of your status between visits; anticoagulant therapy *must* be carefully monitored.
- Tell your doctor if you're planning a trip (even a short one), because changes in diet and environment can affect your medication.
- Don't forget to mention your anticoagulant therapy to your dentist. Even *minor* surgical procedures require consultation with your physician.

- Stay away from all foods that are high in vitamin K; they can interfere with the anticoagulant activity of the drug.

35. Antidepressants (mood elevators)

WHAT THEY DO

- Assist the passage of nerve impulses through brain circuits.
- Stabilize the chemical balance of the brain tissue.

WHAT THEY'RE USED FOR

- To relieve clinical mental depression and depression that can occur with anxiety.
- To treat enuresis (bedwetting).
- Phobias.

POSSIBLE SIDE EFFECTS

For tricyclic antidepressants: Constipation, dizziness, dry mouth, headache, craving for sweets, nausea, rapid heartbeat, fatigue, weight gain, diarrhea, excessive perspiration, heartburn, increased sensitivity to sunlight, vomiting.

For monoamine oxidase (MAO) inhibitor antidepressants: Constipation, difficult urination, lightheadedness, drowsiness, dry mouth and fatigue, chills, impotence, hallucinations, weight gain, increased sensitivity to sunlight, insomnia, muscle twitching, nightmares, shakiness. (For foods and vitamins that can help combat side effects, see section 54.)

SOME BRAND NAMES	GENERIC NAME	SPECIAL NOTES
ADAPIN	*Doxepin*	tricyclic
ELAVIL	*Amitriptyline*	tricyclic
LIMBITROL	*Chlordiazepoxide, amitriptyline*	combination benzodiazepine and tricyclic

SOME BRAND NAMES	GENERIC NAME	SPECIAL NOTES
LUDIOMIL	Maprotiline hydrochloride	not a tricyclic or an MAO
MARPLAN	Isocarboxazid	MAO inhibitor
NARDIL	Phenelzine	MAO inhibitor
NORPRAMIN	Desipramine hydrochloride	tricyclic
PARNATE	Tranylcypromine sulfate	MAO inhibitor
SINEQUAN	Doxepin hydrochloride	tricyclic
TOFRANIL	Imipramine hydrochloride	tricyclic
VIVACTIL	Protriptyline hydrochloride	tricyclic

FOODS THAT CAN INCREASE EFFECTIVENESS

whole wheat, oatmeal, peanuts, dark green leafy vegetables, eggs, cantaloupe (contain vitamins and minerals which aid in fighting depression)

FOODS THAT CAN DECREASE EFFECTIVENESS

carbohydrates, junk foods, sugar (can cause Vitamin B_1 loss and contribute to depression). *For anyone taking MAO inhibitors, it is essential to avoid the following foods which can cause severe hypertension, stroke—even death:* aged cheese, aged meat, pods of broad beans, beer, wines, pickled herring, yogurt, liver, yeast extract, excessive amounts of caffeine and chocolate, ripe bananas, soy sauce, anchovies, avocado, and sour cream (be sure to ask your doctor for a *complete* listing)

CAUTIONS

- The safety of MAO inhibitors during pregnancy and lactation has not been established, so discuss the risks with your physician.
- Antidepressants must often be taken for *several weeks* before effects are felt, so never double up on a medication in the hope of making it more effective faster.
- MAO inhibitors should not be given to anyone with a history of congestive heart failure or abnormal liver function.
- The most serious reaction to MAO inhibitors is a dangerous elevation of blood pressure, which is why foods with a high tyramine content (see above) should be avoided, along with cold, hay fever, and weight-reducing medications—for at least two weeks after discontinuing drug!
- MAO inhibitors can affect blood sugar levels and alter diabetic test results.
- Adverse drug reactions can occur if MAOs and tricyclic antidepressants are given with any other antidepressants or within 10 days after discontinuing other antidepressant therapy.

NATURE'S PHARMACY

- Vitamins B_1, B_6, and B_{12} can help improve mental attitude.
- Choline aids in sending nerve impulses to the brain and produces a soothing effect.
- Calcium helps your nervous system, especially in impulse transmission.
- Magnesium can aid in fighting depression.
- Manganese can reduce nervous irritability.
- L-tryptophan is a natural relaxant which is also used as an antidepressant. It is an amino acid present in many protein foods (especially turkey) that can pass rapidly from the stomach to the nerve centers of the brain.
- L-phenylalanine, another amino acid found in many protein foods, is a natural antidepressant that works in a fashion similar to tryptophan. But L-phenylalanine can raise blood pressure.

(For a quick reference list of foods that contain the vitamins and minerals mentioned, see section 55.)

MY ADVICE

- Even if you think that your antidepressant therapy isn't working, don't stop. Check with your doctor and reduce your drug intake gradually to avoid a relapse or severe withdrawal symptoms.
- If you're going to have any surgery (including dental surgery), it's important to inform the doctor that you are using or have used antidepressants within the last 2 weeks.
- In case no one has mentioned it, "recreational" drugs (specifically cocaine) can cause *serious* adverse reactions if you're taking MAO inhibitors.
- Some people prefer to take pills with carbonated beverages, but these—as well as grape juice—can decrease the potency of tricyclic antidepressants.
- Though alcohol is not prohibited with tricyclics, you're more likely to develop stomach problems if you drink while on these drugs.
- L-tryptophan, which can be purchased OTC at natural food stores, is a wonderful natural relaxant. A 1 g. dose (approximately the content of a turkey dinner) can reduce the time it takes to fall asleep—without altering normal sleep cycles! (To be effective, tryptophan supplements should be taken with water or juice—no protein.)
- L-phenylalanine, a natural "upper," can raise spirits and energy if taken in 500 mg. to 1 gram doses, upon arising, with water or juice (no protein).

36. Antidiabetics, Oral

WHAT THEY DO

- Help reduce the amount of sugar present in the blood, usually by stimulating the body to produce its own *insulin*.

WHAT THEY'RE USED FOR

- Certain types of sugar diabetes (diabetes mellitus).
- For diabetics who do not require *insulin* shots.

POSSIBLE SIDE EFFECTS

Diarrhea, headache, indigestion, loss of appetite, nausea, skin rash, dark urine, itching, jaundice, light-colored stools, sore throat. (For foods and vitamins that can help combat side effects, see section 54.)

SOME BRAND NAMES	GENERIC NAME	SPECIAL NOTES
DIABINESE	Chlorpropamide	takes up to 1 week to give full benefit
ORINASE	Tolbutamide	takes up to 1 week to give full benefit; headache, heartburn, & stomach upset are not uncommon
TOLINASE	Tolazamide	when transferring from other oral antidiabetic drugs, no transition period is necessary

FOODS THAT CAN INCREASE EFFECTIVENESS

brewer's yeast, poultry, eggs, spinach, asparagus, cabbage, celery, fish liver oil, fresh fruit (contain nutrients that aid body in proper utilization of food)

FOODS THAT CAN DECREASE EFFECTIVENESS

carbohydrates, refined sugar, colas, alcohol (can worsen condition since diabetes is characterized by an insufficiency of insulin to process carbohydrates)

CAUTIONS

- Consult your doctor before taking antidiabetic medications if you're pregnant, think you're pregnant, or are a nursing mother.
- Do *not* take an oral antidiabetic if you're on other medications (especially anticoagulants, *aspirin,* diuretics, MAO inhibitors, *cortisones,* seizure or heart medicines) without consultation with your doctor.
- You might have to be switched to *insulin* if you develop a severe infection, need surgery, or become pregnant.
- Beware of OTC cough, cold, and diet medications. (See sections 138-143.)

NATURE'S PHARMACY

- B vitamins help promote the digestion of carbohydrates, which is important because diabetes is characterized by an insufficiency of *insulin* to process carbohydrates.
- Niacin can help increase energy by aiding the body in the proper utilization of food.
- Chromium can work as an important deterrent for diabetes.
- Manganese and zinc can aid in the treatment of diabetes.

(For a quick reference list of foods that contain the vitamins and minerals mentioned, see section 55.)

MY ADVICE

- Because diabetics lose more vitamin C than nondiabetics, daily supplementation of the vitamin is recommended (1,000–3,000 mg. daily); but before starting any regimen, check with your doctor or a nutritionally-oriented physician (see section 167).
- Don't ignore exercise. It's an important factor in diabetes treatment and can determine your *insulin* needs.
- Raw vegetables, seeds, fruits, and nuts can reduce your need for *insulin.* (See sections 138–143.)

- If symptoms of low blood sugar appear (unusual tired-
  ness or weakness, cold sweats, excessive hunger, rapid
  pulse), eat or drink something containing sugar (orange
  juice, honey candy) immediately—and call your doctor.
- Never skip meals!

37. Antidiarrheals

WHAT THEY DO

- Slow the overactive stomach and bowel to relieve diarrhea.

WHAT THEY'RE USED FOR

- Symptomatic relief of diarrhea

POSSIBLE SIDE EFFECTS

Constipation, nausea, dryness of skin and mouth, flushing,
swelling of the gums, decrease in urination, blurred vision,
numbness of hands or feet, rapid heartbeat. (For foods and
vitamins that can help combat side effects, see section 54.)

SOME BRAND NAMES	GENERIC NAME	SPECIAL NOTES
DONNAGEL-PG	Kaolin, pectin, belladonna alkaloids, opium	available in some states without Rx
IMODIUM	Loperamide	not for all forms of diarrhea; can worsen certain kinds of bowel or stomach disease; not for children under 12
LOMOTIL	Diphenoxylate & atropine	

SOME BRAND NAMES	GENERIC NAME	SPECIAL NOTES
PAREGORIC	Opium preparations	
PAREPECTOLIN	Kaolin, pectin, & paregoric	available in some states without Rx

FOODS THAT CAN INCREASE EFFECTIVENESS	FOODS THAT CAN DECREASE EFFECTIVENESS
scraped apple, ripe banana, yogurt, carob flour, strained carrots, small amounts of fiber-rich bran (can act as natural antidiarrheals)	fats, fried foods, milk, chocolate (can worsen attacks of diarrhea)

CAUTIONS

- Do not take medicine longer than directed, as it may become habit-forming.
- If you're pregnant, think you might be pregnant, or are a nursing mother, do not take an antidiarrheal without consulting your doctor.
- Beware of antidiarrheals if you are now taking any CNS (central nervous system) depressants, such as antihistamines, barbiturates, pain-killers, sedatives, tranquilizers, or tricyclic antidepressants. (Kaopectate and plain Kaolin/pectin—only preparations can be taken safely.)
- These medicines can cause drowsiness, so use caution if driving or operating machinery.
- If you suffer from colitis, emphysema, asthma, bronchitis, prostate problems, gallbladder disease, high blood pressure, kidney or liver ailments, over- or underactive thyroid, check with your doctor before taking this type of medication.

NATURE'S PHARMACY

- *Lactobacillus acidophilus* yogurt can help control diarrhea caused by antibiotic regimens.

- Niacin can ease some attacks of diarrhea.
- Carrots are one of the best natural antidiarrheals.

(For a quick reference list of foods that contain the vitamins and minerals mentioned, see section 55.)

MY ADVICE

- Always try natural remedies first before resorting to prescription antidiarrheals.
- Carrots can work wonders! There are at least six antifungal substances in carrots, which means that in some cases of fungus-caused diarrheas, the carrots can help kill off the offending agent (much as an antibiotic would). Also carrots are high in vitamin A, which is an anti-infective vitamin. They are also high in fiber.
- Milk, for people who have or develop an intolerance to it, can cause diarrhea—even in such small amounts as used in coffee or tea. Additives in milk substitutes can also cause diarrhea.

38. Antihistamines (cold and allergy medicines)

WHAT THEY DO

- Dry up secretions of nose, throat, and eyes.
- Relieve or prevent the symptoms of hay fever and other types of allergies by reducing the allergic response of tissues.

WHAT THEY'RE USED FOR

- Allergies
- Nausea
- Sleep difficulties
- Colds
- Dizziness
- Motion sickness
- Tremors and stiffness in Parkinson's disease

POSSIBLE SIDE EFFECTS

Dry nose, mouth, and throat, drowsiness, itching, rash, chills, increased perspiration, rapid heartbeat, blurred vision, tingling of hands and feet, ringing in ears, difficulty in urination, constipation, diarrhea, disturbed coordination, nervousness. (For foods and vitamins that can help combat side effects, see section 54.)

SOME BRAND NAMES	GENERIC NAME	SPECIAL NOTES
ACTIFED	Triprolidine & pseudoephedrine	also a decongestant
ATARAX	Hydroxyzine	also used in treatment of nervous and emotional disorder
BENADRYL	Diphenhydramine	
DIMETAPP	Brompheniramine, phenylephrine, & phenylpropanolamine	also a decongestant
DRIXORAL	Dexbrompheniramine & pseudoephedrine	also a decongestant
NALDECON	Phenylpropanolamine, phenylephrine, phenyltoloxamine, & chlorpheniramine	also a decongestant
ORNADE	Chlorpheniramine, phenylpropanolamine, & isopropamide	also a decongestant
PERIACTIN	Cyproheptadine hydrochloride	also an anti-cholinergic with sedative effects

FOODS THAT CAN INCREASE EFFECTIVENESS	*FOODS THAT CAN DECREASE EFFECTIVENESS*
citrus fruits, juices, watercress, green leafy vegetables, bananas (contain natural antihistaminic properties)	chocolate, refined sugars, colas, alcohol (can worsen allergy symptoms and deplete body of needed stress vitamins)

CAUTIONS

- It is unwise to take an antihistamine, even one that's OTC, unless specifically directed to do so by a physician if you have an overactive thyroid, ulcers, high blood pressure, heart disease, or prostate problems.
- If you are pregnant, thinking of becoming pregnant, or are a nursing mother, do not take any antihistamine (even an OTC preparation) without consulting your doctor.
- Beware of combining an antihistamine with pain-killers, tricyclic antidepressants, seizure medicines, barbiturates, and any sort of tranquilizer—also with any other anti-histamine.
- Consult your doctor before taking an antihistamine if you have taken an MAO inhibitor within the previous 2 weeks.
- Keep in mind that antihistamines can cause drowsiness—even in recommended and prescribed dosages!

NATURE'S PHARMACY

- Vitamin C can aid in the prevention and treatment of symptoms of the common cold and many allergic reactions.
- Potassium can help in allergy treatments.
- And once again, yes, chicken soup!

(For a quick reference list of foods that contain the vitamins and minerals mentioned, see section 55.)

MY ADVICE

- If you find that the antihistamine you're taking upsets your stomach, try taking it with food or a glass of milk.

- You'll lose the effectiveness of "long-lasting" type antihistamines if you crush or chew them. They should be swallowed whole.
- An antihistamine that is prescribed for motion sickness won't help once the sickness is upon you. Take the medication at least 30 minutes before you travel. In fact, 1 to 2 hours before is even better. And *even better*, as far as I'm concerned, is leaving the antihistamines for allergies and taking 100 mg. of vitamin B complex the night before and the morning of your trip.

39. Antihyperlipidemics (cholesterol reducers)

WHAT THEY DO

- Decrease fatty substances in the blood—namely cholesterol and triglycerides.

WHAT THEY'RE USED FOR

- Prevention of hardening of the arteries (blood vessels coming from the heart).
- Decrease risk of heart attack and stroke.

POSSIBLE SIDE EFFECTS

Nausea, diarrhea, heartburn, vomiting, dizziness, impotence, loss of hair, itching, rash, increased appetite, sores in mouth, fatigue. (For foods and vitamins that can help combat side effects, see section 54.)

SOME BRAND NAMES	GENERIC NAME	SPECIAL NOTES
ATROMID-S	*Clofibrate*	
CHOLOXIN	*Dextrothyroxine sodium*	
NICOBID	*Timed release nicotinic acid*	may be better tolerated than tablet form

SOME BRAND NAMES	GENERIC NAME	SPECIAL NOTES
NICOLAR	Niacin	may cause flushing, itching and stomach upset

FOODS THAT CAN INCREASE EFFECTIVENESS	FOODS THAT CAN DECREASE EFFECTIVENESS
eggplant, onions, garlic, yogurt, soybeans (can help to naturally lower cholesterol)	liver, fatty foods, fried foods, sugar, coffee (can raise cholesterol levels)

CAUTIONS

- This drug can increase your risk of cancer, liver disease, inflammation of the pancreas, and gallstones.
- Don't take this drug if you are pregnant, trying to become pregnant, or are a nursing mother. (ATROMID-S can be harmful to your baby for up to several months *before* you become pregnant.)
- Avoid taking this medication if you're now using anticoagulants or diuretics.

NATURE'S PHARMACY

- Vitamin B_{15} (pangamic acid) has been found to lower blood cholesterol levels.
- Decreases in blood cholesterol levels have occurred with supplements of vitamin C.
- Decreasing your sugar intake can help to lower triglycerides and cholesterol.
- Choline helps prevent cholesterol buildup.
- Vitamin F (unsaturated fatty acids—linoleic, linolenic, and arachidonic) aids in preventing cholesterol deposits in the arteries.
- Another member of the vitamin B complex group, inositol, can help lower cholesterol levels.

- Niacin helps reduce cholesterol. (It's sold as the prescription drug NICOLAR!)
- Zinc can promote a decrease in cholesterol deposits.

(For a quick reference list of foods that contain the vitamins and minerals mentioned, see section 55.)

MY ADVICE

- An antihyperlipidemic should be a last resort drug, used only after diet, weight loss, and exercise have failed to lower your cholesterol and triglyceride levels.
- If you're watching your cholesterol levels, a meal of light-meat turkey is a good choice, especially since no more than 300 mg. of cholesterol a day are recommended for the average person. Three ounces of light-meat turkey have only 67 mg. of cholesterol (dark meat has 75 mg.).
- Watch out for turkey liver! One cup chopped has about 839 mg. cholesterol!
- And if you haven't heard enough reasons to stop smoking, here's one more: it raises cholesterol levels.
- Stress can also raise cholesterol levels, but B vitamins and L-tryptophan are a better answer than tranquilizers.
- Women using birth control pills should be aware that it raises their levels of cholesterol, while posing other risks (see section 66).

40. Antihypertensives (high blood pressure reducers, Vasodilators) and Diuretics ("water pills")

WHAT THEY DO

- Stimulate nerve receptors that inhibit stress.
- Dilate blood vessels.
- Increase flow of urine.

WHAT THEY'RE USED FOR

- Lower blood pressure
- Congestive heart failure

- Any condition where excess fluids must be eliminated
- Kidney malfunction
- Cirrhosis of liver

POSSIBLE SIDE EFFECTS

Nausea, diarrhea, constipation, headache, tingling of toes and fingers, dry mouth, rash, blurred vision, dizziness, muscle spasms, fatigue, loss of sexual desire, sexual dysfunction, mental depression.

(For foods and vitamins that can help combat side effects, see section 54.)

SOME BRAND NAMES	GENERIC NAME	SPECIAL NOTES
ALDACTAZIDE	*Spironolactone & hydrochlorothiazide*	a combination of two diuretic agents; minimizes potassium loss
ALDACTONE	*Spironolactone*	can cause breast enlargement in men; a diuretic that does *not* cause potassium loss
ALDOMET	*Methyldopa*	can cause impotence; an antihypertensive
ALDORIL	*Methyldopa & hydrochlorothiazide*	can cause impotence; an antihypertensive-diuretic
APRESOLINE	*Hydralazine hydrochloride*	can cause angina attacks; an antihypertensive
BLOCADREN	*Timolol maleate*	a beta-adrenergic blocker

SOME BRAND NAMES	GENERIC NAME	SPECIAL NOTES
CAPOTEN	Captopril	an antihypertensive
CATAPRES	Clonidine	an antihypertensive
DIURIL	Chlorothiazide	thiazide diuretic
DYAZIDE	Triamterene & hydrochlorothiazide	a combination of 2 diuretics; may cause increase or loss of potassium
ENDURON	Methyclothiazide	thiazide diuretic
ESIDRIX	Hydrochlorothiazide	thiazide diuretic
HYDRODIURIL	Hydrochlorothiazide	thiazide diuretic
HYGROTON	Chlorthalidone	an anithypertensive-diuretic; sensitivity reactions may occur in patients with a history of allergy or bronchial asthma
INDERAL	Propranolol hydrochloride	a cardiovascular drug that controls heart rhythm as well as lowers blood pressure; a beta-adrenergic blocker
LASIX	Furosemide	diuretic; may cause sensitivity to sunlight
LOPRESSOR	Metoprolol tartrate	same as INDERAL above
MIDAMOR	Amiloride hydrochloride	potassium-conserving diuretic
MINIPRESS	Prazosin hydrochloride	an antihypertensive

SOME BRAND NAMES	GENERIC NAME	SPECIAL NOTES
REGROTON	Reserpine & chlorthalidone	thiazide diuretic-antihypertensive; may cause sensitivity to sunlight and mood changes
SALUTENSIN	Reserpine & hydroflumethiazide	thiazide diuretic-antihypertensive; potentiates action of other antihypertensives
SER-AP-ES	Hydralazine, hydrochlorothiazide, & reserpine	thiazide diuretic-antihypertensive; can cause nightmares and mood changes
TENORMIN	Atenolol	a cardiovascular drug compatible with thiazide diuretics

FOODS THAT CAN INCREASE EFFECTIVENESS	FOODS THAT CAN DECREASE EFFECTIVENESS
garlic, green leafy vegetables, yeast, wheat germ (can help lower blood pressure)	salted foods, luncheon meats, frankfurters, corned beef, ketchup, soy sauce, mustard (high in sodium and can cause water retention and elevated blood pressure)

CAUTIONS

- If you are pregnant or a nursing mother, discuss the risks involved in taking any antihypertensive or diuretic.
- Before having any surgery (including dental), be sure your doctor knows the medication you're on.

- Don't take any antihypertensive or diuretic if you have heart, kidney, or liver disease—or a history of mental depression—without consulting your doctor.
- Some antihypertensives can cause a buildup of potassium, while others (particularly thiazide diuretics) deplete it. Be sure you know which your drug is doing and adjust your diet and supplements accordingly.

NATURE'S PHARMACY

- Vitamin B_6 (pyridoxine) works as a natural diuretic.
- Potassium assists in reducing blood pressure.
- Alfalfa is a natural diuretic.
- Garlic can act as a vasodilator and substantially lower blood pressure.

(For a quick reference list of foods that contain the vitamins and minerals mentioned, see section 55.)

MY ADVICE

- Many high blood pressure pills cause dizziness when you stand up suddenly, so avoid sudden changes in posture.
- Some diuretics cause a zinc and potassium loss, so make sure you're eating enough bananas, citrus fruits, melons, tomatoes, green leafy vegetables, and unsalted sunflower seeds.
- Don't overdo a good thing. Too much potassium can cause hyperkalemia (excessive potassium in the blood). Regular blood tests can make sure you're on the right nutritional track.

41. Anti-inflammatories/Antiarthritics (for inflammations & arthritis)

WHAT THEY DO

- Help relieve swelling, joint pain, stiffness, and fever.

WHAT THEY'RE USED FOR

- Arthritis
- Tendinitis
- Skin problems
- Bursitis
- Joint pains or spasms
- Spinal pain
- Asthma
- Severe allergies

POSSIBLE SIDE EFFECTS

Diarrhea, nausea, water retention, mental confusion, headache, irritability, unusual weight gain, drowsiness, bloating, ringing in the ears, blurred vision, skin rash, mental depression. (For foods and vitamins that can help combat side effects, see section 54.)

SOME BRAND NAMES	GENERIC NAME	SPECIAL NOTES
BUTAZOLIDIN	Phenylbutazone	
CLINORIL	Sulindac	see Section 119
INDOCIN	Indomethacin	see Section 119
MECLOMEN	Meclofenamate sodium	for optimum benefit, 2–3 weeks of treatment may be required
MEDROL	Methylprednisolone	a steroid; may cause blood sugar levels to rise in diabetics; may cause stomach bleeding
MOTRIN	Ibuprofen	see Section 119
NALFON	Fenoprofen calcium	see Section 119
NAPROSYN	Naproxen	see Section 119

SOME BRAND NAMES	GENERIC NAME	SPECIAL NOTES
TOLECTIN DS	*Tolmetin sodium*	see Section 119
VANCERIL	*Beclomethasone*	a steroid; used with an inhaler; can help prevent asthma attack, but will not help one that has already begun; may cause stomach bleeding

FOODS THAT CAN INCREASE EFFECTIVENESS	FOODS THAT CAN DECREASE EFFECTIVENESS
raw fruits and vegetables, nuts, whole wheat, potatoes, fish, poultry (contain vitamins and minerals that can help alleviate distress due to inflammation)	salty foods, luncheon meats, refined carbohydrates, alcohol (can worsen inflammatory conditions)

CAUTIONS

Antiarthritic and anti-inflammatory drugs are potent and can cause serious side effects, such as perforated ulcers, gastrointestinal hemorrhage, and liver and kidney damage, if not taken precisely as directed.

- Don't take this medication if you are pregnant, trying to become pregnant, or are a nursing mother.
- This medicine can be dangerous if you are allergic to *aspirin,* or have any medical problems such as ulcers (even sores or white spots in the mouth); heart, liver, or kidney disease; stomach problems; or asthma.
- Anti-inflammatories can react adversely with blood-thinners, oral diabetes medicine, *tetracyclines,* other arthritis medicines, and iron preparations. Be sure your doctor knows what you're now taking!

- Avoid *aspirin* and alcohol while on this type of medication.
- If you are taking another steroid medicine for asthma along with VANCERIL, don't stop the other without consulting your doctor, even if your asthma seems better.
- Don't stop taking any steroid medicine without consulting your doctor; unsupervised withdrawal can have devastating effects on the body.

NATURE'S PHARMACY

- Vitamin B_6 (pyridoxine) can reduce night muscle spasms, leg cramps, hand numbness, and certain forms of neuritis.
- Vitamin B_{12} (cobalamin) and iron can be helpful in treating the anemia that may accompany arthritis.
- Biotin aids in easing muscle pains.
- Vitamin C is necessary to prevent capillary walls in the joints from breaking down and causing swelling and pain.
- Vitamin D is helpful in properly utilizing calcium and phosphorus, which are necessary for strong bones.

(For a quick reference list of foods that contain the vitamins and minerals mentioned, see section 55.)

MY ADVICE

- You can reduce stomach upset by taking these drugs with food or a full (8 oz.) glass of milk.
- Don't take BUTAZOLIDIN ALKA (buffered *phenylbutazone*) with vitamin supplements that contain iron or special iron preparations. Take them 1 to 2 hours apart or you can prevent the iron from being absorbed.
- Many cases of arthritis can be avoided or alleviated by eliminating gluten from the diet. It's worth a 1-month trial period.
- If you are taking MEDROL (*methylprednisolone*), be sure to inform the doctor in charge if you are having any skin tests, immunization, or surgery.
- Supplements of vitamin C and pantothenic acid in dosages of 1,000 mg. daily are important for arthritis sufferers.

42. Antinauseants (Antiemetics)

WHAT THEY DO

- Depress responses that cause nausea.

WHAT THEY'RE USED FOR

- Motion sickness
- Nausea
- Dizziness
- Morning sickness
- Vomiting
- Diseases of inner ear
- Disturbances in the sense of balance

POSSIBLE SIDE EFFECTS

Drowsiness, dry mouth, blurred vision, tremors. (For foods and vitamins that can help combat side effects, see section 54.)

SOME BRAND NAMES	GENERIC NAME	SPECIAL NOTES
ANTIVERT	Meclizine	
ATARAX	Hydroxyzine	an antihistamine used also in the treatment of nervous disorders (see section 38)
BENDECTIN	Doxylamine & pyridoxine	can produce palpitations, vertigo, and irritability; now off the U.S. market
DRAMAMINE	Dimenhydrinate	also an anti-histamine; no Rx necessary, but see section 38 for general cautions

SOME BRAND NAMES	GENERIC NAME	SPECIAL NOTES
TIGAN	*Trimethobenzamide hydrochloride*	may contribute, in combination with viral illnesses, to development of Reye's syndrome in children

FOODS THAT CAN INCREASE EFFECTIVENESS	FOODS THAT CAN DECREASE EFFECTIVENESS
wheat bran, wheat germ, cantaloupe, milk, eggs, beef (NOTE: These foods are high in antinauseant B vitamins but are to be eaten while on medication, *not* when nauseated.)	spicy, rich, fatty, or fried foods; coffee (can worsen feelings of nausea)

·CAUTIONS

- BENDECTIN, formerly prescribed for morning sickness in pregnancy, is now off the market because studies have shown that high dosages can cause birth defects in laboratory animals.
- If you are a nursing mother, antinauseants may pass into the breast milk and adversely affect your infant.
- These medications will increase the effects of alcohol and other drugs that slow down the nervous system—including some dental anesthetics.
- If you're taking large amounts of *aspirin,* signals that would·indicate you're taking too much (ringing in the ears) can be masked by antinauseants.

NATURE'S PHARMACY

- Vitamin B_1 (thiamine) and vitamin B_6 (pyridoxine) alleviate nausea and can help prevent motion and morning

sickness. (Many morning sickness preparations that doctors prescribe include vitamin B_6!)
- Niacin can reduce the unpleasant symptoms of vertigo in Meniere's syndrome.
- Vitamin P (C complex, citrus bioflavonoids, rutin, hesperidin) helps in the treatment of dizziness due to disease of the inner ear.

(For a quick reference list of foods that contain the vitamins and minerals mentioned, see section 55.)

MY ADVICE

- Before leaving yourself open to a variety of unwanted side effects, I'd advise trying vitamin B_6 without added drugs as a preventive for morning and motion sickness. Since vitamin B_1 can also help, and vitamins B_1, B_2, and B_6 are most effective when taken in a balanced formula, I'd advise taking a B-complex formula (100 mg.) at night and in the morning, with juice or milk, upon arising.
- Ginger root capsules, available in natural food stores, taken 3 times daily are nature's best anti-morning sickness remedy.

43. Antispasmodics/Anticholinergics ("stomach and cramp pills")

WHAT THEY DO

- Relax the digestive system to reduce stomach acid.
- Prevent or control muscle spasms.

WHAT THEY'RE USED FOR

- Ulcers
- Muscle spasms caused by other drugs
- Colitis
- Intestinal cramping
- Treatment of Parkinson's disease

POSSIBLE SIDE EFFECTS

Bloating, nasal congestion, dry mouth, rapid heartbeat, skin rash, mental confusion. (For foods and vitamins that can help combat side effects, see section 54.)

SOME BRAND NAMES	GENERIC NAME	SPECIAL NOTES
BENTYL	*Dicyclomine hydrochloride*	reduces heat tolerance; can cause drowsiness or blurred vision
COGENTIN	*Benztropine mesylate*	might make you sensitive to bright light; don't take within an hour of taking an antacid or diarrhea medicine
COMBID	*Prochlorperazine & isopropamide*	might make you more sensitive to sunlight; PABA sunscreen lotion can help; don't take within 1 hour of taking an antacid or diarrhea medicine
DONNATAL	*Atropine sulfate, hyoscyamine, scopolamine, & phenobarbital*	might cause urine retention
LIBRAX	*Chlordiazepoxide hydrochloride & clidinium bromide*	reduces heat tolerance; can cause drowsiness; should not be taken if you are allergic to benzodiazepines

SOME BRAND NAMES	GENERIC NAME	SPECIAL NOTES
PRO-BANTHINE	*Propantheline*	reduces your tolerance of heat (use with caution during hot weather and exercise) and could cause heat stroke; don't take within 1 hour of taking an antacid or diarrhea medicine

FOODS THAT CAN INCREASE EFFECTIVENESS	FOODS THAT CAN DECREASE EFFECTIVENESS
lean meats, white meat of poultry, whole grains, eggs, nuts, alfalfa (contain nutrients that can alleviate gastrointestinal distress)	fried and fatty foods, refined carbohydrates, coffee, alcohol (can worsen intestinal cramps and spasms)

CAUTIONS

- These drugs should not generally be taken if you suffer from glaucoma; myasthenia gravis; heart, lung, kidney, or blood diseases; or any sort of intestinal blockage.
- If you are pregnant, trying to become pregnant, or are a nursing mother, discuss with your doctor the risks involved in taking this type of drug.
- Do not start on an antispasmodic/anticholinergic regimen if you've been taking MAO inhibitors within the previous 2 weeks.
- Avoid taking antihistamines, pain-killers, tranquilizers, narcotic medicines, or antidepressants with this medication.

NATURE'S PHARMACY

- All the B vitamins aid digestion, helping to metabolize carbohydrates and assimilate protein and fat.

- Niacin helps promote a healthy digestive system and alleviates gastrointestinal disturbances.
- Alfalfa and raw cabbage juice has been used successfully in treatment of a variety of stomach ailments and ulcerous conditions.

(For a quick reference list of foods that contain the vitamins and minerals mentioned, see section 55.)

MY ADVICE

- Dry mouth is a common side effect with anticholinergics and antispasmodics, but chewing on bits of ice can help. (When away from home, you'll find sugarless gum will work.)
- If you want a delicious way to improve your digestion, try papaya. It's not only great-tasting, but it actually helps you digest food! The alpha and beta papain enzymes in papaya break down protein; the chymopapain enzyme helps break down *all* food.
- Before rushing to the pharmacy, you might want to try peppermint for your abdominal cramps. A cup of cool peppermint tea can work wonders.

44. Anti-uric acid/Anti-gout drugs

WHAT THEY DO

- Lower uric acid levels in the body by either increasing uric acid excretion or inhibiting its formation.

WHAT THEY'RE USED FOR

- Gout
- Certain types of cancer
- Increasing the effectiveness of some antibiotics
- Psoriasis

POSSIBLE SIDE EFFECTS

Nausea, stomach pain, headache, loss of appetite, skin rash (see "Special Notes" below), itching, diarrhea, drowsiness, frequent urination, sore gums. (For foods and vitamins that can help combat side effects, see section 54.)

SOME BRAND NAMES	GENERIC NAME	SPECIAL NOTES
ANTURANE	Sulfinpyrazone	
BENEMID	Probenecid	may cause false results on diabetic sugar tests
ZYLOPRIM	Allopurinol	differs from other anti-gout drugs by inhibiting the formation of uric acid rather than increasing its excretion; should be discontinued at first sign of skin rash or any sign of adverse reaction!

FOODS THAT CAN INCREASE EFFECTIVENESS	FOODS THAT CAN DECREASE EFFECTIVENESS
cherries, berries, fruits, fruit juices (can help reduce uric acid)	organ meats, condiments, alcohol, spinach, lentils, asparagus, mushrooms, concentrated sweets, fried foods (high purine foods which can trigger attacks of gout)

CAUTIONS

• Do not take any of these medications if you're pregnant,

trying to become pregnant, or are a nursing mother, without discussing the risks involved with your physician.

- Before taking any anti-uric acid drug, inform your doctor if you have any history of ulcers, blood, or kidney disease.
- Do not take ZYLOPRIM (*allopurinol*) if you or any member of your immediate family has idiopathic hemochromatosis (a disease that prevents the body from properly metabolizing iron)!
- Don't take supplemental vitamin C while taking ZYLOPRIM; it increases the possibility of kidney stones.
- Inform your doctor of all other medications you're taking. (Antibiotics, anticoagulants, diuretics, *aspirin*, and diabetes medications can, in particular, interact adversely.)

NATURE'S PHARMACY

- Magnesium can help prevent calcium deposits, kidney and gallstones.
- Phosphorus can aid in reducing the pain of gouty arthritis.
- Yeast can help reverse gout and ease the aches and pains of neuritis.
- Pantothenic acid promotes proper metabolic functioning of the cells.

(For a quick reference list of foods that contain the vitamins and minerals mentioned, see section 55.)

MY ADVICE

- Drink water! Lots of it! With any of these medications it's advisable to drink at least 10 full (8 oz.) glasses a day to help prevent the formation of kidney stones.
- If *allopurinol* upsets your stomach, take it *after* meals; other medications can be taken with food or milk.
- Since these medications are used primarily to prevent attacks of gout and rarely relieve one that has already started, try eating cherries. Cherries and cherry juice, according to Dr. Ludwig W. Blau in *Texas Reports on Biology and Medicine,* help metabolize uric acid and prevent the crystallization of it, which causes gouty pain.

- Because low-purine diets, which exclude certain foods and are often prescribed to avoid triggering attacks of gout (see section 125), normally lack vitamin E and the B-complex vitamins, I'd advise supplements: Vitamin E (dry form) 200 to 400 IU and vitamin B-complex 100 mg. 1 to 3 times daily.

45. Appetite suppressants/Anorexics ("diet pills")

WHAT THEY DO

- Stimulate the central nervous system and suppress appetite.

WHAT THEY'RE USED FOR

- Control of obesity
- Narcolepsy

POSSIBLE SIDE EFFECTS

Euphoria, irritability, restlessness, nervousness, insomnia, constipation or diarrhea, dizziness, dry mouth, headache, increased urination, palpitations, elevated blood pressure. (For foods and vitamins that can help combat side effects, see section 54.)

SOME BRAND NAMES	GENERIC NAME	SPECIAL NOTES
DEXEDRINE	Dextroamphetamine sulfate	an amphetamine with high potential for drug dependence
DIDREX	Benzphetamine	an amphetamine-related drug with high potential for dependence

SOME BRAND NAMES	GENERIC NAME	SPECIAL NOTES
FASTIN	*Phentermine hydrochloride*	tolerance develops within a few weeks; high potential for dependence; not recommended for patients with even *mild* hypertension
IONAMIN	*Phentermine resin*	an amphetamine-related drug with high potential for dependency; may decrease the hypotensive activity of ISMELIN
PRELUDIN	*Phenmetrazine hydrochloride*	an amphetamine-related drug with high potential for dependency
TENUATE	*Diethylpropion hydrochloride*	an amphetamine-related drug with high potential for dependency

FOODS THAT CAN INCREASE EFFECTIVENESS	FOODS THAT CAN DECREASE EFFECTIVENESS
kelp, eggs, apple cider vinegar (contain nutrients which can help in weight reduction)	refined carbohydrates, sugars, fried and fatty foods (contain empty calories which undermine purpose of medication)

CAUTIONS

- Avoid any type of "diet pill" if you are pregnant, thinking of becoming pregnant, or are a nursing mother.

(Amphetamines increase the chance of birth defects if taken in the early months of pregnancy; though this hasn't been shown with other types of appetite suppressants, there's always a risk.)

- Don't take these medicines if you have any medical problems (particularly diabetes, epilepsy, glaucoma, heart disease, high blood pressure, or an overactive thyroid).
- Be aware, if you are a diabetic, that your *insulin* requirement may be altered because of these drugs.
- Don't start therapy with this type of medication if you're taking MAO inhibitors, or have done so within the previous 2 weeks.
- Don't mix these drugs with caffeine, other stimulants, tranquilizers, or antihypertension medication.
- When you stop taking this type of medication, you might suffer a variety of side effects, from fatigue to mental depression.
- Keep in mind that all these drugs can be extremely habit forming.

NATURE'S PHARMACY

- Vitamin B_6 helps in weight reduction by acting as a natural diuretic.
- Vitamin B_{12} aids in properly utilizing fats, carbohydrates, and protein, and also increases energy.
- Vitamin E can also work as a diuretic.
- Vitamin F (unsaturated fatty acids—linoleic, linolenic, and arachidonic) promotes weight reduction by burning saturated fats.
- Inositol helps in the redistribution of body fat.
- Iodine can help you with dieting by regulating the thyroid gland which burns fat.
- Potassium is important in helping to dispose of body wastes.
- Water before meals is one of the safest appetite suppressants you can use.
- Kelp, because of its natural iodine content, can aid in weight reduction by normalizing the thyroid gland.

(For a quick reference list of foods that contain the vitamins and minerals mentioned, see section 55.)

MY ADVICE

- Appetite suppressants are *not* alternatives to diet and exercise. Their appetite-reducing effect is only temporary, and the pills should be used only as short-term measures (no longer than 12 weeks).
- If you feel that your family doctor doesn't understand your dieting needs, contact a bariatrician, who specializes in the field. (For the name of one in your area, write to the American Society of Bariatric Physicians, Suite 300, 5200 South Quebec, Englewood, Colorado 80111.)
- If you're taking diet pills in conjunction with a low-carbohydrate diet, weight might not be all that you're losing. Chances are your potassium level is down, which can cause weakness and poor reflexes. Make sure you're taking a high-potency multivitamin and multimineral preparation to avoid this. (For further information on dieters' drugs, see sections 76–84.)

46. Cardiovascular preparations—Anti-anginals, Vasodilators (heart medicines)

WHAT THEY DO

- Reduce blood pressure and chest pain.
- Dilate arteries and capillaries to improve circulation.
- Control the rhythm of the heart.
- Increase the force of heart contractions and help it to pump.

WHAT THEY'RE USED FOR

- Heart failure
- Angina pectoris
- Preventives and treatments for various other heart conditions
- Heart disease

- Abnormal heart
- High blood pressure
- Mitral valve disease

POSSIBLE SIDE EFFECTS

Nausea, headache, flushing, weakness, loss of appetite, decreased sex drive, constipation or diarrhea, dizziness. (For foods and vitamins that can help combat side effects, see section 54.)

SOME BRAND NAMES	GENERIC NAME	SPECIAL NOTES
CORGARD	Nadolol	beta-blocker; used primarily in treatment of angina and hypertension; causes slowing of heart rate; may cause blood sugar levels of diabetics to fall and mask signs of hypoglycemia
CYCLOSPASMOL	Cyclandelate	a vasodilator; should be used with caution in patients with glaucoma
INDERAL	Propranolol	beta-blocker; same as for CORGARD above; also known as "the confidence pill" because it reduces trembling, sweaty palms, etc. due to temporary nervousness

SOME BRAND NAMES	GENERIC NAME	SPECIAL NOTES
ISORDIL	Isosorbide dinetrate	most effective as a *preventive* for anginal attacks
LANOXIN	Digoxin	improves strength of the heart; tablets or capsules might look like other medications you take, so mark these *distinctly*
NITRO-BID	Nitroglycerin	after taking medicine you may get a headache that lasts a short while; do not take any analgesic without consulting your doctor
NITROL	Nitroglycerin	same as above
NITROSTAT	Nitroglycerin	same as above
NORPACE	Disopyramide phosphate	an anti-arrhythmic; may cause or worsen congestive heart failure; can produce severe low blood pressure
PAVABID	Papaverine hydrochloride	a vasodilator; should be used with caution in patients with glaucoma

SOME BRAND NAMES	GENERIC NAME	SPECIAL NOTES
PERSANTINE	*Dipyridamole*	contains FD&C Yellow No. 5 (*tartrazine*) which may cause allergic reactions
QUINIDINE SULFATE	*Quinidine sulfate*	slows overactive heart; is potentiated by potassium
SORBITRATE	*Isosorbide dinitrate*	contains FD&C Yellow No. 5 (*tartrazine*) which may cause allergic reactions

FOODS THAT CAN INCREASE EFFECTIVENESS	*FOODS THAT CAN DECREASE EFFECTIVENESS*
citrus fruits, green leafy vegetables, bananas, fish (contain nutrients which help promote a healthy cardiovascular system)	refined carbohydrates, saturated fats, coffee (can raise blood pressure, cholesterol levels, and essentially undermine benefits of above-mentioned medicines)

CAUTIONS

- If you're pregnant, thinking of becoming pregnant, or are a nursing mother, discuss the risks involved in taking a beta-adrenergic blocking agent (LOPRESSOR, COR-GARD, INDERAL) with your doctor.
- The use of *propranolol* during pregnancy can lower the heart rate of a newborn infant.
- Before taking any of these drugs, be sure to inform your physician of any medical problems you might have (particularly emphysema; diabetes; heart, liver, blood, or

kidney disease) and any medications you are taking or have taken within the previous 2 weeks.

- Discuss with your doctor how much exercise you can do, since many of these medications mask the pain and warning signals of overexertion.
- Sublingual (under-the-tongue) *nitroglycerin* tablets, if not stabilized, can lose their potency before the marked expiration date because of repeated patient usage, opening of bottle under different moisture and temperature conditions, and so on. (Most new *nitroglycerin* medicines *are* stabilized, but check with your pharmacist anyway.)
- *Never put other pills in the same bottle with nitroglycerin*; they'll weaken the *nitroglycerin*'s effect.
- Do not take PERSANTINE to relieve an angina attack. This drug is a preventive and too slow-acting to be of help once an attack has begun. Ask your doctor about *nitroglycerin*.

NATURE'S PHARMACY

- Vitamin B_1 helps keep your heart functioning normally.
- Vitamin B_{15} can aid in relieving the symptoms of angina.
- Vitamin C lowers the incidence of blood clots in veins.
- Vitamin E helps in preventing and dissolving blood clots, as well as reducing blood pressure.
- Vitamin F (unsaturated fatty acids—linoleic, linolenic, and arachidonic) helps in combating heart disease.
- Niacin increases blood circulation and helps reduce high blood pressure.
- Chromium helps in the prevention of certain heart ailments by promoting lower blood pressure.
- Magnesium can help prevent heart attacks by promoting a healthier cardiovascular system.
- Zinc can act as a preventive for heart attacks by decreasing cholesterol deposits.

(For a quick reference list of foods that contain the vitamins and minerals mentioned, see section 55.)

MY ADVICE

- If you're taking beta-blockers (INDERAL, CORGARD, LOPRESSOR), bundle up in cold weather. These drugs tend to decrease circulation and make you more sensitive to cold.
- If you're an angina sufferer and you feel that your present medication is not working as successfully as it should, ask your doctor about the new combination therapy of beta-blockers and calcium-blockers. It seems that the beta-blocker *propranolol* (INDERAL) combined with the calcium-blocker *nifedipine* (PROCARDIA) works more effectively than either drug by itself. But be aware that combining another calcium-blocker *verapamil* (ISOPTIN, CALAN) with a beta-blocker is *not* advised. According to the FDA, *verapamil* should be used alone.
- If you have a heart problem, the right diet is essential (see section 135). And it's not only what you eat but how you eat it that matters. It's better for you and your heart to eat smaller portions frequently (5 or 6 light meals) than to eat less frequently and have one or two large meals.
- Walking is great for the circulation. If taking time out for a therapeutic constitutional doesn't appeal to you, why not just park your car ¼ to ½ mile further away than usual from your home or office? The extra walking won't seem like exercise at all—and you'll be surprised at how much weight you can lose in a year.
- No matter what medication you're taking, the worst thing you can do for your heart is just sit around and think about it!

47. Decongestants and expectorants

WHAT THEY DO

- Act on the small blood vessels to shrink swollen mucous membranes in the nose, permitting easier drainage and freer breathing.
- Unclog throat, bronchial tubes, or lungs, making it easier to cough up congested material.

WHAT THEY'RE USED FOR

- Colds
- Allergies
- Coughs

POSSIBLE SIDE EFFECTS

Dryness of nose, mouth, and throat, headache, palpitations, nervousness, constipation/diarrhea, dizziness, drowsiness, skin rash, nausea, loss of appetite. (For foods and vitamins that can help combat side effects, see section 54.)

SOME BRAND NAMES	GENERIC NAME	SPECIAL NOTES
ACTIFED-C EXPECTORANT	Codeine phosphate, triprolidine hydrochloride, pseudoephedrine hydrochloride, glyceryl guaiacolate	should not be used in the treatment of asthma
AMBENYL EXPECTORANT	Codeine sulfate, bromodiphenhydramine hydrochloride, ammonium chloride, potassium guaiacolsulfonate	FDA feels there is a lack of substantial evidence that this drug has the effect purported
BENYLIN COUGH SYRUP	Diphenhydramine hydrochloride, ammonium chloride, sodium citrate	may cause excitability, especially in children
DIMETANE EXPECTORANT-DC	Brompheniramine maleate, guaifensin, phenylephrine, phenylpropanolamine, & codeine	
PHENERGAN EXPECTORANT	Promethazine hydrochloride	can cause photosensitivity

SOME BRAND NAMES	GENERIC NAME	SPECIAL NOTES
PHENERGAN EXPECTORANT w/CODEINE	Promethazine hydrochloride & codeine phosphate	can cause photosensitivity; may cause constipation & heart-pounding
TUSSIONEX	Resin complexes of hydrocodone & phenyltoloxamine	can potentiate effects of alcohol and any drugs that slow down the nervous system
TUSS-ORNADE SPANSULES	Caramiphen edisylate, chlorpheniramine maleate, isopropamide, iodide, phenylpropanolamine hydrochloride	should not be used for children under 12

FOODS THAT CAN INCREASE EFFECTIVENESS	FOODS THAT CAN DECREASE EFFECTIVENESS
garlic, citrus fruits & juices, wheat germ (can aid in treatment of coughs, colds, and allergies)	refined carbohydrates, sugar (can deplete body of needed illness-fighting nutrients)

CAUTIONS

- If you are pregnant, trying to become pregnant, or are a nursing mother, consult your doctor before taking any of these medications. Although none have been proven conclusively to cause problems, there is always a risk.
- Do not take any of these medications if you're on any other drugs (especially anticonvulsants, antihypertensives, and ulcer medications) without consulting a doctor.
- CNS (central nervous system) depressants (barbiturates, pain-killers, antidepressants, other antihistamines) can interact adversely with these medications.

- If you are taking large amounts of *aspirin* (for arthritis), warning effects of overdose might be masked by these drugs.
- Do not give these medications to infants.
- These medicines may be habit forming.

NATURE'S PHARMACY

- Vitamin A can build resistance to respiratory infections.
- Vitamin C aids in treatment of colds, allergies, and accompanying symptoms.
- Vitamin P (C complex, citrus bioflavonoids, rutin, hesperidin) increases the effectiveness of vitamin C and helps build resistance to infection.
- Potassium aids in the treatment of allergies and accompanying symptoms.
- Garlic can alleviate bronchial congestion.

(For a quick reference list of foods that contain the vitamins and minerals mentioned, see section 55.)

MY ADVICE

- Try taking garlic (it's available in easy-to-swallow perles). These caps contain valuable garlic oils that can break up bronchial congestion and leave no after-odor on the breath because they dissolve in the lower digestive tract, not the stomach.
- Remember warm liquids are better than cold ones for relieving stuffy noses and congestion from coughs. (Hot chicken soup really works!)
- Before rushing out to fill a prescription, why not try a natural cough syrup: Cook 6 chopped white onions and ½ cup of honey in the top of a double boiler, over low heat, for 2 hours. Strain. Take 1 to 2 tablespoons every two or three hours. (The remedy works best when warm.)

48. Laxatives

WHAT THEY DO

- Provide bulk which stimulates evacuation.
- Encourage bowel movements by helping liquids mix into the stool to prevent dry hard masses and straining.

WHAT THEY'RE USED FOR

- Relief of constipation during pregnancy and after child-birth (only bulk-forming and emollient laxatives should be used for this; check CAUTIONS below).
- Before or after surgery
- To counteract constipation caused by other medicines
- To supply stool samples for diagnosis
- For medical conditions where straining should be avoided

POSSIBLE SIDE EFFECTS

Stomach cramps, gas, diarrhea, nausea, fatigue. (For foods and vitamins that can help combat side effects, see section 54.)

SOME BRAND NAMES	GENERIC NAME	SPECIAL NOTES
CASCARA SAGRADA	Cascara sagrada	stimulant type; action slowed if taken with food
CHRONULAC	Lactulose	used for long-term treatment; Rx necessary
COLACE	Docusate sodium	emollient type (stool softener)
COLOGEL	Methylcellulose	bulk-forming type
EPSOM SALTS	Magnesium sulfate	saline type; fast-acting, not for long-term use

SOME BRAND NAMES	GENERIC NAME	SPECIAL NOTES
EX-LAX	Phenolphthalein	stimulant type
FEEN-A-MINT	Phenolphthalein	stimulant type
FLETCHER'S CASTORIA	Senna	stimulant type
METAMUCIL	Psyllium hydrophilic mucilloid	bulk-forming type
MITROLAN	Calcium polycarbophil	bulk-forming type
MUCILOSE	Psyllium mucilloid, psyllium seed, psyllium	bulk-forming type
NEOLOID	Castor oil	stimulant type; results usually in 2 to 6 hours
NUJOL	Mineral oil	lubricant type; large doses may cause leakage from rectum
SAL HEPATICA	Sodium phosphate, effervescent sodium phosphate	saline type; fast-acting; not recommended for extended use
SURFAK	Docusate calcium	emollient type (stool softener)

FOODS THAT CAN INCREASE EFFECTIVENESS	FOODS THAT CAN DECREASE EFFECTIVENESS
whole grains, bran, fruit, water, green leafy vegetables, licorice, sesame seeds (can help promote easier bowel movements)	hard cheeses, refined carbohydrates (can contribute to constipation)

CAUTIONS

- If you are pregnant, avoid saline laxatives (EPSOM SALTS, SAL HEPATICA) and laxative preparations containing mineral oil, castor oil, or sodium.
- Never take a laxative if you have any symptoms of appendicitis, such as abdominal pain (particularly on lower right side) with tenderness to pressure.
- Avoid taking a laxative without consulting your doctor if you are presently using birth control pills, taking antibiotics, anticoagulants, heart medicines, other laxatives, or antacids.
- Lubricant laxatives can interfere with your body's ability to absorb nutrients and inhibit absorption of the oil-soluble vitamins A, D, E, and K.
- Many laxatives contain large amounts of sodium, which elevate blood pressure and cause water retention.
- Do not take laxatives if you have any medical problems without getting specific instructions from your doctor.
- Laxatives can reduce the effects of other medicines, so take them at least 2 hours apart. (This is particularly true for lubricant laxatives taken too closely with birth control pills and anticoagulants.)
- Don't take a laxative if it gives you a rash!

NATURE'S PHARMACY

- Vitamins B_1, B_2, B_6, and B_{12} aid in assimilation of protein fats and carbohydrates to promote a healthy digestive system.
- Vitamin C can act as a natural laxative.
- Potassium helps dispose of body wastes.
- Water helps prevent constipation.
- Acidophilus keeps the intestines clean and aids in preventing constipation.
- Alfalfa is a natural laxative.
- Bran, which is also available as a food supplement in concentrated tablet form, provides a good amount of soft bulk that speeds bowel movements.

(For a quick reference list of foods that contain the vitamins and minerals mentioned, see section 55.)

MY ADVICE

- Don't resort to a laxative just because you miss a bowel movement for a day or two. (There's no rule that bowels must be moved every 24 hours.)
- The best treatment for constipation is proper diet, adequate amounts of roughage, such as bran, whole grain cereals, raw fruits, and green leafy vegetables, along with plenty of liquids (at least six 8-oz. glasses daily).
- Harsh laxatives can not only rob the body of nutrients, but also cause rebound constipation and laxative dependency. A reliable natural remedy is:

    2 tbsp. unprocessed bran flakes daily

    3–9 bran tablets daily

    1 tbsp. acidophilus liquid 3 times daily

    (If necessary, a vegetable laxative and stool softener can be used for a short time.)
- The juice of a lemon mixed in a glass of hot water ½ hour before breakfast is another effective natural laxative. (Licorice, boiled as tea, will also work.)

49. Oral contraceptives, estrogens, and progestogens (birth control pills and sex hormones)

WHAT THEY DO

- Change the hormone balance of the body to prevent pregnancy.
- Aid normal sexual development of women.
- Promote necessary development of milk-producing glands and regulate the menstrual cycle.

WHAT THEY'RE USED FOR

- Birth control
- Replacement of hormones after certain types of surgery
- Regulation of menstrual cycle
- Treatment in certain types of breast and prostate cancer
- Menopause therapy
- Hormone tests

POSSIBLE SIDE EFFECTS

Cramps, loss of appetite, nausea, acne, swelling of ankles and feet, tenderness and swelling of breasts, fatigue, brown spots on skin, diarrhea, increased facial and body hair, increased sensitivity to sun, changes in vaginal bleeding (spotting, breakthrough bleeding, prolonged bleeding), skin rash, vaginal discharge, increased blood pressure, yellowing of skin, changes in sex drive, bloating, weight changes. (For foods and vitamins that can help combat side effects, see section 54.)

SOME BRAND NAMES	GENERIC NAME	SPECIAL NOTES
DEMULEN	Ethynodiol diacetate & ethinyl estradiol	oral contraceptive
LO/OVRAL	Norgestrel & ethinyl estradiol	oral contraceptive
NORINYL	Norethindrone & mestranol	oral contraceptive
ENOVID	Norethindrone & mestranol	oral contraceptive
ORTHO-NOVUM	Norethindrone & mestranol	oral contraceptive
OVRAL	Norgestrel & ethinyl estradiol	oral contraceptive
OVULEN	Ethynodiol diacetate & mestranol	oral contraceptive
DIETHYLSTIL-BESTROL (DES)	Diethylstilbestrol	estrogen (see section 69)
PREMARIN	Conjugated estrogens	estrogen; should not be used during pregnancy

SOME BRAND NAMES	GENERIC NAME	SPECIAL NOTES
PROVERA	Medroxyprogesterone acetate	progestogen; depression might recur to a serious degree in patients who were former depressives
NORLUTATE	Norerthindrone acetate	progestogen

FOODS THAT CAN INCREASE EFFECTIVENESS	FOODS THAT CAN DECREASE EFFECTIVENESS
brewer's yeast, liver, milk, eggs, citrus fruits (contain nutrients that promote a healthy reproductive system)	refined carbohydrates, coffee (can increase loss of already depleted B vitamins)

CAUTIONS

- Do not take any of these medications if you're pregnant, think you're pregnant, or are a nursing mother. (Estrogens and/or progestogens can cause birth defects if taken during pregnancy.) If you think you've become pregnant while on one of these drugs, stop using it immediately and contact your doctor!
- If you smoke, be aware that taking the Pill (combination of estrogen and progestin) makes you more susceptible to heart attacks, strokes, high blood pressure, and formation of hazardous blood clots in the veins.
- Avoid oral contraceptives if you have a medical history of cancer, diabetes, asthma, epilepsy; heart, liver, or thyroid disease; or are presently taking anticoagulants, tranquilizers, or sedatives.
- These medications can alter your blood-clotting ability, so tell your doctor (or dentist) what drug you're taking before having any surgery.
- Wait at least three months after taking oral contraceptives before trying to become pregnant.

- Your body requires time to adjust to oral contraceptives, so use other contraceptive methods for at least three weeks after starting a Pill regimen to prevent pregnancy.
- The Pill neutralizes normal vaginal acids, making women who use it more susceptible to gonorrhea and other vaginal infections.

NATURE'S PHARMACY

- Vitamin B_{12}, as part of a B-complex, alleviates discomfort during and just prior to menstruation.
- Vitamin C helps diminish hot flashes and can aid in reducing excessive menstrual bleeding.
- Vitamin E helps prevent blood clots, discomforts of menopause, and also aids in the prevention of miscarriages.
- Folic acid improves lactation.
- Vitamin K aids in reducing excessive menstrual flow.
- Niacin eases the severity of migraine headaches.
- Vitamin P (C complex, citrus bioflavonoids, rutin, hesperidin) helps relieve hot flashes in menopausal women when taken in conjunction with vitamin C.
- Calcium aids in relieving menstrual cramps.
- Selenium can alleviate hot flashes and menopausal distress.
- Zinc helps promote menstrual regularity.
- Ginseng can relieve hot flashes during menopause.

(For a quick reference list of foods that contain the vitamins and minerals mentioned, see section 55.)

MY ADVICE

- If you are on the Pill or taking either estrogen or progestin alone, you're playing dangerous games with your nutrition. Many Pill users are seriously deficient in folic acid, as well as vitamins B_1, B_2, B_6, B_{12}, C, E, and essential minerals such as zinc and magnesium.
- If you're taking oral contraceptives and you're depressed, it's not surprising. Your need for B_6 (necessary for normal tryptophan metabolism) is fifty to 100 times a non-Pill-user's requirements. Supplements are definitely in order. I'd suggest the following regimen:

- A high-potency multiple vitamin with chelated minerals 1–2 times daily
- Vitamin C, 1,000 mg., 1 to 3 times daily
- Folic acid, 800 mcg., 1 to 3 times daily
- Zinc (chelated), 50 mg., 1 to 3 tablets daily
- Vitamin B_{12}, 500 mcg., 2 to 3 times daily
- Vitamin B_6, 50 mg., 2 to 3 times daily

- If you go off the Pill in order to become pregnant, do NOT take vitamin A supplements, or eat vitamin-A-rich foods (see section 55), but do increase the folic acid in your diet. Too much vitamin A and too little folic acid have, in this instance, been associated with birth defects.
- If you have any menopause-type distress, vitamin E supplements, 100–400 mg. daily (start low and increase gradually), can make you feel much better.
- Taking these medications is nothing to lose your hair over, but it sometimes happens. The best way to counteract it is to add zinc and a good vitamin B-complex to your diet.
- Before rushing into ERT (estrogen replacement therapy) to alleviate menopause-related distress, see section 69 and 70.
- Keep in mind that there are other forms of birth control less hazardous to your health, especially if you're over 35 and a smoker. Why not talk them over with your doctor?

50. Tranquilizers, sedatives, relaxants, barbiturates, and hypnotics

WHAT THEY DO

- Tranquilizers are sedatives that decrease anxiety and other psychic unrest without putting the patient to sleep.
- Relaxants are tranquilizers that act particularly on muscles to relieve physical and mental "tightness."
- Sedatives, hypnotics, and barbiturates are designed primarily to produce sleep.

WHAT THEY'RE USED FOR

- Anxiety
- Muscle spasms
- Tension
- Insomnia
- Depression
- Psychic disorders
- Acute emotional distress

POSSIBLE SIDE EFFECTS

Drowsiness, dizziness, confusion, nausea, diarrhea or constipation, dry mouth, palpitations, elevated or lowered blood sugar levels, blurred vision, slurred speech, irregular heart rhythms, high or low blood pressure, weight gain, urine retention, nightmares, sweating, hallucinations, drug tolerance/dependence. (For foods and vitamins that can help combat side effects, see section 54.)

SOME BRAND NAMES	GENERIC NAME	SPECIAL NOTES
ATIVAN	*Lorazepam*	a benzodiazepine; used for short-term relief of anxiety symptoms; peak effects occur 2 hours after administration
BUTISOL SODIUM	*Butabarbital sodium*	a barbiturate; sedative hypnotic; onset of action is approximately 30 minutes—duration of action is 5–6 hours
CENTRAX	*Prazepam*	a benzodiazepine; tranquilizer used for short-term relief of anxiety symptoms

SOME BRAND NAMES	GENERIC NAME	SPECIAL NOTES
COMPAZINE	Prochlorperazine	tranquilizer for control of severe anxiety and severe nausea and vomiting
DALMANE	Flurazepam hydrochloride	a benzodiazepine; sedative; used for treatment of various types of insomnia; an additive effect may occur if alcohol is consumed the day *following* use of DALMANE; might take 2 or 3 days to achieve full effect
DORIDEN	Glutethimide	an hypnotic; high potential for abuse; combined with codeine it's stronger than heroin, ten times more addicting, and considered deadlier (see section 97)
FLEXERIL	Cyclobenzaprine	relieves skeletal muscle spasms without interfering with muscles
HALDOL	Haloperidol	major tranquilizer used in the management of psychic disorders

SOME BRAND NAMES	GENERIC NAME	SPECIAL NOTES
LIBRIUM	Chlordiazepoxide	a benzodiazepine; tranquilizer for relief of anxiety as well as withdrawal symptoms of acute alcoholism; can cause vivid dreams
LUDIOMIL	Maprotiline hydrochloride	tranquilizer/ antidepressant; for anxiety related to depression
MELLARIL	Thioridazine hydrochloride	tranquilizer for anxiety and depression; used for treatment of severe behavioral problems in children; can cause breast enlargement
MEPROBAMATE	Meprobamate	tranquilizer for treatment of nervousness or tension
MILTOWN	Meprobamate	tranquilizer for treatment of nervousness or tension
PARAFON FORTE	Acetaminophen, chlorzoxazone	muscle-skeletal relaxant
PHENOBARBITAL	Phenobarbital	a barbiturate; hypnotic, sedative, anticonvulsant

SOME BRAND NAMES	GENERIC NAME	SPECIAL NOTES
RESTORIL	Temazepam	a benzodiazepine; hypnotic; for treatment of insomnia
SERAX	Oxazepam	a benzodiazepine; tranquilizer for treatment of anxiety associated with depression and other causes; should be used cautiously by the elderly and anyone for whom a drop in blood pressure could cause cardiac complications
STELAZINE	Trifluoperazine hydrochloride	tranquilizer; should be used with caution by angina patients
THORAZINE	Chlorpromazine	tranquilizer; also used to treat nausea, vomiting, and continuing hiccups; the ability to cough is reduced by this medication
TRANXENE	Chlorazepate	a benzodiazepine; tranquilizer; quickly appears in bloodstream; not recommended for use in depressive neuroses

SOME BRAND NAMES	GENERIC NAME	SPECIAL NOTES
TRIAVIL	*Amitriptyline hydrochloride, perphenazine*	tranquilizer/ antidepressant; can cause changes in menstrual cycle, black tongue, sensitivity to sunlight
VALIUM	*Diazepam*	a benzodiazepine; tranquilizer/muscle relaxant; narcotics, barbiturates, and antidepressants potentiate its effects
XANAX	*Alprazolam*	a benzodiazepine; tranquilizer for treatment of anxiety; not recommended for treatment of psychotic patients

FOODS THAT CAN INCREASE EFFECTIVENESS	FOODS THAT CAN DECREASE EFFECTIVENESS
milk, turkey, fish, green leafy vegetables (contain nutrients which can act as natural tranquilizers and relaxants)	refined carbohydrates, chocolate, cola, foods seasoned with MSG (deplete stress vitamins and can worsen psychotic conditions)

CAUTIONS

- Do not use these medications if you're pregnant, trying to become pregnant, or are a nursing mother, without consulting your doctor about the risks involved.

- Be sure to inform your doctor if you have any medical problems (especially epilepsy; any lung, kidney, or liver disease; or a history of mental illness).
- These medications can cause loss of alertness, so know how you react to them before you drive or operate machinery!
- Many of these drugs can interact adversely with the ulcer medication TAGAMET.
- Beware of mixing tranquilizers with other tranquilizing medications, pain-killers, and antidepressants.
- In small doses, barbiturates (PHENOBARBITAL) may increase your reaction to painful stimuli.
- Barbiturates should not be relied on to relieve pain—in fact, they're usually ineffective in producing sleep in the presence of severe pain.
- Avoid eating large mouthfuls of food, because tranquilizers such as COMPAZINE and THORAZINE reduce the ability to cough.
- THORAZINE should be used with caution if you're going to be exposed to extreme heat, which could foster drug accumulation.
- Pregnant women who take PHENOBARBITAL late in their pregnancy may jeopardize the sexual development of their male offspring by causing reduced levels of the male hormone testosterone.
- Never mix any of these drugs with alcohol—the combination can be *deadly!* (See sections 156, 157.)
- And remember, these drugs have a high potential for dependence and can be habit forming.

NATURE'S PHARMACY

- Vitamin B_1 is known as the "morale vitamin" because of its beneficial effects on the nervous system and mental attitude.
- Vitamin B_6 helps prevent various nervous disorders and alleviates nausea.
- Vitamin B_{12} can relieve irritability and help in the maintenance of a healthy nervous system.
- Choline aids in eliminating nervous or "twitchy" feelings.

- All the B vitamins and vitamin C can help the body fight stress.
- Niacin is necessary for a healthy nervous system.
- Calcium aids your nervous system, especially in impulse transmission.
- Magnesium can help in fighting depression.
- Manganese can reduce nervous irritability.
- Zinc is important for all brain functions, and has been used in the treatment of schizophrenia.
- Pantothenic acid and inositol can be effective alternatives to sleeping pills.
- L-tryptophan is one of nature's top tranquilizers.

MY ADVICE

- Tranquilizers and other medicines can be bad combinations. For example, taking an analgesic like DARVON with a tranquilizer can result in tremors and serious mental confusion. The same thing can happen by combining a sedative with a simple OTC antihistamine.
- If you take antacids and still want your tranquilizer to be effective, make sure you take it at least two hours before the antacid.
- If you're taking DALMANE (*flurazepam*) on a regular basis for an extended period of time, it's wise to check in with your doctor every month. (With other drugs of this type, every four months is sufficient.)
- Always be on the alert for an overdose. Warning signs are extreme weakness, difficult breathing, severe drowsiness, and unusually slow heartbeat. Call for emergency help at once. (Also, if you experience hangovers or mental confusion while taking any of these medications, you might need a prescription change, so contact your doctor.)
- Before resorting to sedatives or hypnotics, why not try a glass of warm milk (calcium) and an open-face turkey sandwich. (Turkey is a great source of tryptophan!)

51. Ulcer medicines

Most ulcer medications are antispasmodics and anticholinergics, and can be found listed in section 43. It should be noted though that TAGAMET (*cimetidine*), a relatively new drug and one of the most popularly prescribed medications for ulcers in the United States, is not an anticholinergic. It is the first in a new class of drugs called histamine H2 receptor antagonists, and it aids in the treatment of ulcers by inhibiting gastric acid secretions.

If you are pregnant, planning to become pregnant, or are a nursing mother or have a kidney disease, do not take this medication without discussing the risks involved with your doctor. Also, be aware that TAGAMET can interact adversely with anticoagulants (see section 34) and benzodiazepines (ATIVAN, CENTRAX, DALMANE, LIBRIUM, RESTORIL, SERAX, TRANXENE, VALIUM).

TAGAMET can cause dizziness and mental confusion, so it should be used with caution if you drive or operate machinery. It can also cause an increase in breast size or breast soreness in men (though this particular side effect is usually only temporary).

It often takes several days (sometimes weeks) for TAGAMET to effectively relieve stomach pain, so you might want to discuss the possibility of taking an antacid along with the medication with your doctor. For advice on foods and supplements, see section 43.

52. What you should know about other popular prescriptions

ANTICONVULSANTS

DILANTIN (*phenytoin*), which is ranked among the top twenty most prescribed drugs in the United States, is used most often to control a variety of convulsions or seizures. Common side effects are swollen or bleeding gums (1,000 mg. of vitamin C complex three times daily helps), uncontrolled rolling of the eyes, and unstable walking.

If you are on any other medications, are—or are planning to become—pregnant, or if you're a nursing mother or are about to have surgery (including dental), it is *essential* that you consult with your doctor. (*Phenytoin* has been found in breast milk in amounts large enough to produce undesirable effects in nursing infants.)

Be warned that alcoholic beverages are capable of making

this medicine more potent than is desirable, so check with your doctor before partying. DILANTIN can also alter the blood sugar level of diabetics.

ANTIDYSKINETICS

ARTANE (*trihexyphenidyl*) is a widely prescribed drug for the treatment of Parkinson's disease. Like COGENTIN (see section 43), which is also used to treat Parkinson's, the drug's primary action is improving muscle control and reducing the stiffness indicative of the disease.

These medicines will become less effective if taken within an hour of taking an antacid or diarrhea medication. ARTANE and COGENTIN also have a variety of side effects, the most common being dizziness, a feeling of bloatedness, dry mouth, headache, and rapid pulse. (See section 54 for foods and vitamins that can help.) In addition, they may cause your eyes to become uncomfortably sensitive to light and reduce your body's tolerance to heat. To avoid heat stroke, be careful not to become overheated during exercise or hot weather, and use caution if taking hot baths or saunas.

BRONCHIAL DILATORS

BRETHINE (*terbutaline sulfate*), CHOLEDYL (*oxtriphylline*), QUIBRON (*theophylline-guaifenesin*), SLO-PHYLLIN GYROCAPS (*theophylline, anhydrous*), THEO-DUR (*theophylline, anhydrous*) are bronchial dilators used in the treatment of asthma, emphysema, chronic bronchitis and other lung diseases to relax the smooth muscle of bronchial airways and pulmonary blood vessels to allow easier breathing.

These drugs should not be used if you are pregnant, thinking of becoming pregnant, if you are a nursing mother, or have any existing medical problems, without consulting your doctor about the risks involved. You should also check with your doctor before taking these medications if you've ever had an adverse reaction to *aminophylline, dyphylline, oxtriphylline, theobromine, theophylline* or caffeine!

Common side effects for these medicines are headaches, nervousness, stomach cramps and nausea (see section 54 for natural remedies that can help). If mental confusion, excessive thirst, frequent urination or unusual fatigue occur, it could be a sign of overdose and you should contact your doctor immediately.

While on this type of medication, it's advisable to stay away from all caffeine-containing drinks (tea, coffee, cola, cocoa) because their stimulant effects can be increased, often uncomfortably so. And if you're troubled by excess mucus, milk products should also be avoided.

DERMATOLOGICALS

HYTONE (*hydrocortisone*), KENALOG (*triamcinolone*), LIDEX (*fluocinonide*), MYCOLOG (*nystatin, neomycin sulfate, gramicidin & triamcinolone acetonide*), SYNALAR (*fluocinolone*) and VALISONE (*betamethasone*) are topical cortisone-like medicines which are used to treat skin problems (itching, swelling, redness, etc), and fall into the general category of medications called steroids. Prolonged use of any of these drugs is not recommended since they can be absorbed through the skin. For this reason it is unwise to use these medicines if you are pregnant, planning to become pregnant, a nursing mother, or have an infection at the treatment site, without discussing your situation with a doctor. (It's also very important to tell your doctor if you've ever had an allergic reaction to any other cortisone-type medication!)

Unless you've been specifically directed to do so, do not bandage the area that's being treated. This can increase the amount of medicine that's being absorbed through the skin and lead to unwanted side effects. (If using these medicines on an infant's diaper area, it's best not to put rubber or plastic pants on the child.)

These medicines are contraindicated for many types of viral and bacterial infections and therefore should be used only for the particular skin problems for which they were prescribed.

Keep in mind, too, that iodine can worsen a dermatological condition, so avoid highly salted foods (pickles, processed cheeses, etc.) and any others that use iodized salt.

GERIATRICS

HYDERGINE (*ergoloid mesylates*) is used to treat mental confusion, depression, and other general symptoms of incipient senility in older persons. This medicine essentially improves blood circulation to the brain, but is not useful in treating migraine headaches and should not be taken by anyone who is allergic to other ergot alkaloids (ERGOSTAT, SANSERT). If using the sublingual (under-the-tongue) form of this medication, do not smoke or drink while the tablet is dissolving.

Side effects are rare, but soreness beneath the tongue, dizziness upon arising, and nausea can occur. Any discomfort, though, should be brought to the attention of your doctor.

If you're taking this medicine, don't expect immediate results. HYDERGINE often takes several weeks to be really effective. Also, this medication can lessen your ability to adjust to the cold, so bundle up and don't expose yourself to cold temperatures for an extended period of time.

Choline, a member of the B-complex family, is one of the few substances able to penetrate the blood-brain barrier (which ordinarily protects the brain against variations in the daily diet) and go directly into brain cells to produce a chemical that aids memory. A supplement of choline and inositol, 1,000 mg., would be advisable to take daily.

HEMORRHOIDAL PREPARATIONS

ANUSOL-HC (*hydrocortisone, bismuth, benzyl benzoate, peruvian balsam,* and *zinc oxide*) is a rectal, cortisone-like medication. It is used to alleviate the itching and swelling of hemorrhoids and other rectal problems. Available as a cream or suppository, it should not be used for longer than the time period for which it has been prescribed as it is a steroid and can be absorbed to an unwanted degree through the rectal tissues. (It can affect growth and should not be given to children unless treatment is specifically prescribed—and monitored—by a doctor.)

Before using this medication, be sure to inform your doctor if you're pregnant, thinking of becoming pregnant, are a nursing mother, or are allergic to any hydrocortisone products or other rectal medicines. This medicine shouldn't be used if you have an infection at the treatment site, and your doctor should be informed immediately if signs of irritation occur after starting treatment. For how to handle a hemorrhoid naturally, see section 117.

OPHTHALMIC SOLUTIONS

- Though applied topically, these drugs may be absorbed systemically and enter the bloodstream.
- TIMOPTIC (*timolol maleate*), used to reduce intraocular (within the eyeball) pressure, is a beta-adrenergic blocker and can cause the same unwanted side effects, such as low blood pressure, congestive heart failure, slow heartbeat, dizziness and difficult breathing; it also can mask the warning signals for *insulin*-dependent diabetics. (See cautions indicated for INDERAL and LOPRESSOR in section 40.)

SODIUM SULAMYD (*sulfacetamide sodium*) is used for treatment of bacterial eye infections, such as conjunctivitis, but should not be used by anyone who is—or suspects that he or she is—sensitive to sulfonamides (GANTRISIN, BACTRIM, SEPTRA, GANTANOL).

NEOSPORIN OPHTHALMIC (*polymyxin B, bacitracin & neomycin*), used for short-term treatment of external eye infections caused by organisms susceptible to its antibiotic ingredients, can cause allergic cross reactions and prevent the use of such antibiotics as *kanamycin, paromomycin, streptomycin* and *gentamicin* for the treatment of future infections.

CHLOROMYCETIN (*chloramphenicol*), an antimicrobial eye medication, can cause aplastic anemia with prolonged use.

Vitamins A, D, and calcium can help prevent and treat conjunctivitis. Add more egg yolk, fish, liver, and green and yellow vegetables to your diet and you might not need an ophthalmic prescription at all!

PEDICULICIDES

KWELL (*lindane*) is a shampoo used to kill head, body, and pubic lice (crabs). Though applied topically, *lindane* penetrates human skin and has the potential for CNS (central nervous system) toxicity, especially in infants and children. It should be used *only* as directed—and with caution by pregnant women.

POTASSIUM SUPPLEMENTS

Prescription potassium supplements are necessary for people who have lost too much of the mineral—usually because of illness or use of diuretics—to be replaced by dietary changes or ordinary OTC potassium gluconate supplements (which can contain only 99 mg. of potassium).

Too much potassium, though, can be dangerous and cause hyperkalemia (irregular heartbeat, mental confusion, unexplained anxiety; numbness in hands, feet or lips; difficult breathing), which is why these supplements should not be taken without a doctor's continuing supervision. (In patients with impaired kidney functions, hyperkalemia can cause cardiac arrest.)

The most common side effects of these supplements are nausea, vomiting, diarrhea, and abdominal discomfort. Potassium chloride can be extremely irritating to the stomach, so it's best taken in liquid or dissolvable tablet form. Tablets can be dissolved in juice, but avoid tomato juice if you're on a low-salt diet.

K-LYTE (*potassium chloride*) comes in effervescent tablets, but be aware that it contains saccharin, artificial flavor, and color.

K-TAB (*potassium chloride*) is a slow release tablet and should only be taken if you can't tolerate liquid or effervescent preparations, because it can cause intestinal and gastric ulceration and bleeding. The same is true of MICRO-K and SLOW-K.

Be sure to tell your doctor if you're using salt substitutes— *these already contain potassium!*

THYROID HORMONES

Thyroid supplements are prescribed when blood tests reveal that your thyroid gland is producing insufficient amounts of the hormone necessary for the proper functioning of the body's organ systems (endocrine, nervous, skeletal, reproductive, gastrointestinal).

These supplements should *not* be used in the treatment of

obesity in anyone with a normal thyroid function. In regular doses they will be ineffective; in larger doses (especially when used with certain diet pills) they can be highly toxic!

PROLOID (*thyroglobulin*), which is obtained from purified extract of hog thyroid; SYNTHROID (*levothyroxine sodium*); and THYROID, prepared from defatted, desiccated thyroid glands of edible animals, are the most commonly prescribed.

Many people take thyroid medication for granted, but it can change the effects of other medicines and vice versa. (OTC antihistamines and diet pills should not be taken without consulting your doctor.)

Tell your doctor about any medical problems you have and any medications you're taking (or have recently taken) before filling a prescription for a thyroid supplement. Cholesterol-reducing drugs like QUESTRAN, for example, can inhibit thyroid absorption and should not be taken together.

Kelp can affect your thyroid gland. If you've been using both kelp and a thyroid medicine, you should have your hormone level rechecked. You might need less of the prescription drug than you think.

Large amounts of raw cabbage can cause an iodine deficiency and throw off thyroid production if you have an existing low-iodine intake.

VITAMINS

POLY-VI-FLOR (multiple vitamins and fluoride) and TRI-VI-FLOR (vitamins A, D, C, and fluoride) are pediatric vitamin supplements for children who live in areas where there is not enough fluoride in the drinking water. (Fluoride has been shown to be helpful in reducing cavities.) These preparations work best if taken at bedtime, after the teeth have been brushed. Side effects are rare if the dosage prescribed is correct, but if you notice dark spots on your child's teeth—or if nausea, diarrhea, stomach cramps, or faintness occur—it is a sign of possible overdose and the doctor should be contacted immediately.

STUARTNATAL 1 + 1 TABLETS (multiple vitamins and minerals with one full grain of elemental iron, 200 mg. of calcium, and 1 mg. of folic acid) are prescribed to provide more potent vitamin and mineral supplements throughout pregnancy and the postnatal period. Side effects are rare, though there is the possibility of the folic acid masking symptoms of pernicious anemia and, because the tablets do contain the additive *tartrazine* (FD&C Yellow #5), some women might experience an allergic reaction, particularly if they are sensitive to *aspirin*.

FERROUS SULFATE (inorganic iron) is used to treat iron-deficiency anemia and is often prescribed for women suffering from fatigue due to menstruation or other causes. It should not be taken by anyone with a blood disease such as sickle-cell anemia, hemochromatosis, or thalassemia, and should not be given to children unless a doctor specifically prescribes it for them. If you're taking ferrous sulfate and vitamin E, take them at least eight hours apart. (Ferrous sulfate can destroy vitamin E.) Also, you can inhibit your iron absorption if you consume large quantities of caffeine!

53. Any questions about Chapter VI?

This probably sounds silly, but it seems that whenever I'm on antibiotics, my fingertips hurt. Is there any connection, and can I do anything about it?

If you've been on *tetracycline*, there most likely is a connection. (It's not an uncommon complaint among patients taking the drug.) *Tetracycline* interferes with the body's normal sun-screening properties. Because the nail plate is transparent to ultraviolet light, it can act as a lens and focus light right on the underlying nailbed. In some cases, edema may result, along with a partial detachment of the nail. Nail polish and/or a thick coating of a sun-blocker should help protect your nailbed.

I've been on ELAVIL for the past three years and, though the medication works (mood-wise), the side effects, particularly having a perpetually dry mouth, are depressing. Aren't there any tricyclics that don't cause this?

Unfortunately most tricyclics do have dry mouth as a side effect. But there is a new class of antidepressants called triazolopyridine derivatives, which psychiatrists from the University of Pennsylvania have found comparable to tricyclics, and which have significantly fewer side effects—including dry mouth, blurred vision, and urine retention. The drug to ask your doctor about is DESYREL (*trazodone*).

Are there any new drugs for acne?

ACCUTANE (*isotretinoin*) has recently been given FDA approval for treatment of severe cystic acne which doesn't respond to conventional treatment or antibiotics.

Can you overdose on antihistamines?

You can overdose on any drug! For antihistamines such as *tripelennamine* (PBZ, PYRIBENZAMINE), *diphenhydramine* (BEN-ADRYL, BENYLIN, VALDRENE), *chlorpheniramine* (CHLORA-MATE, UNICELLES, CHLOR-TRIMETON), and others, the probable toxic dose for an adult is anywhere from 1 to 20 grams.

I've been taking aspirin for headaches all my life and have never thought of it as a "drug." Can it really affect other medications I take?

Can it! *Aspirin* is a drug, and a potent one at that, and should never be taken without keeping your other medications in mind. For example:

- It can increase the effectiveness of the antiepileptic drug DILANTIN (*phenytoin*) to a potentially dangerous degree.
- It can suppress the excretion of uric acid and undermine the effectiveness of such drugs as BENEMID and PROBENECID.
- Combined with antidiabetic drugs, it can produce hypoglycemia.
- It can dangerously increase the effectiveness of anticoagulants.
- It can potentiate both the therapeutic *and* toxic effects of MEXATE, a drug used to treat severe psoriasis; and if the toxicity is increased, the results can be fatal.

On the other hand, *aspirin* can potentiate the antibacterial activity of sulfonamides—anti-infective sulfa medicines (e.g. SEPTRA, GANTRISIN, GANTANOL)—as well as lengthen the time that *penicillin* remains in your bloodstream, though it's wise to ask your doctor if this is to your benefit. It's also wise to inform your doctor (or dentist) if you've used *aspirin* within 5 days before any surgical procedure.

Chapter VII

Side Effects

54. Combating side effects with natural foods, supplements, and herbs

No drug is free of side effects! Sometimes you're not aware of them, as in the case of small vitamin losses; other times, as when you're afraid to leave the house because of nausea and diarrhea or dizziness that prevents you from knowing the ceiling from the floor, you're *more* than aware—you're a wreck!

> There's no need to feel like hell while getting well!

The truth is, every time you take a medicine you're bound to get some bad with the good, and if the benefits of a drug outweigh accompanying distress, then side effects are worth it. *But just because side effects can't be avoided doesn't mean they can't be alleviated!* There is no need to feel like hell while getting well.

What follows are some natural solutions to the discomforts of all-too-common side effects of drugs.

IMPORTANT: *Your particular drug therapy might preclude the use of certain foods or vitamins that are suggested. Please be aware that these regimens, along with others in the book, are not prescriptive nor intended as medical advice, and should be discussed with your doctor.*

NAUSEA/VOMITING

- A cup of basil tea, plain or with a little honey, can ease queasiness and help prevent vomiting.
- Chewing on a stick of ginger (or sipping a cup of ginger tea) can also help.
- Vitamin B complex, 100 mg. twice daily, can work as a preventive.

DIZZINESS

- Try grating the rind of ½ lemon (or orange) into a fruit salad every day.
- Be sure you're eating enough green leafy vegetables, beets, egg yolks, milk, liver, cheese, and fish.
- A supplement regimen worth trying is:

Niacin	50–100 mg. 3 times a day
Vitamin E	400 IU 1 to 3 times a day

DIARRHEA

- *Lactobacillus acidophilus* yogurt helps, especially in cases of diarrhea caused by antibiotics. 1 tbsp. acidophilus liquid (or 3 acidophilus tablets) 3 times daily increases the effectiveness.
- Carob flour and bananas are rich in pectin, an effective binder.
- Ironically, adding bran to your diet, which helps in alleviating constipation, can also relieve certain types of diarrhea.

CONSTIPATION

- Unprocessed bran and unprocessed wheat germ 1 tbsp. each daily. (These work better when moistened. Use milk, juice, or soup according to taste.)
- Licorice tea works well as a mild laxative.
- For a more potent laxative herb tea, mix equal parts hedge hyssop leaves, milfoil, American senna leaves, and caraway. Add 1 tsp. to ½ cup water, bring to a boil, and let it cool. Drink twice a day, morning and night.
- A good supplement regimen would be:

Acidophilus liquid   1 tbsp. 3 times daily
Bran tablets   3 to 9 daily

HEADACHE

- Drink a strong cup of peppermint tea, then lie down for 15 to 20 minutes. (This can often work just as effectively as aspirin—and there are NO side effects!)
- A good preventive is vitamin B complex 100 mg. 1 to 3 times daily.

INSOMNIA

- A glass of warm milk at bedtime. (Milk is high in tryptophan, which can work as a natural sedative and tranquilizer.)
- Camomile tea, an old standby that still works.
- A natural supplement regimen that can help is:

Tryptophan tabs 500–667 mg.   3 taken ½ hour before
                              bedtime with water or juice
                              (no protein)

Chelated calcium and
magnesium   1 tab 3 times daily
Vitamin B_6 50 mg. ½ hour before
                              bedtime

ITCHING

- Vitamin E oil applied topically.
- Wheat germ oil can alleviate rectal itching. (Wash af-

- flicted area several times daily with warm water, dry, then apply oil.)
- Dry skin itches are often helped by increasing the vitamin A in your diet (liver, sweet potatoes, carrots) along with some polyunsaturated salad oil (2 tbsp. of corn, safflower, or sunflower oil on a daily salad is sufficient).

LOSS OF APPETITE

- Many people have found the following regimen an effective appetite booster:

Vitamin B-complex	50 mg. with each meal
Vitamin B_{12}	2,000 mcg. (time-release) with breakfast
Organic iron complex (containing vitamin C, copper, liver, manganese, and zinc to help assimilate iron)	1 daily

ECZEMA/SKIN RASHES/DERMATITIS

- Put brewer's yeast into your diet; it's loaded with B vitamins and can work wonders for dermatitis. (Brewer's yeast is available in tablets; take 2 to 6 a day.)
- Vitamin E applied topically.
- A supplement program that beats getting still more prescription medicine is:

Multiple vitamin without minerals (iodine can worsen acne conditions)	1 daily
Vitamin E (dry)	200–400 IU 1 to 2 times daily
Vitamin A (dry)	10,000 IU 1 to 2 times daily for 6 days a week
Chelated zinc	3 times daily with food
Acidophilus liquid	3 times daily

ANXIETY/NERVOUSNESS

- An herbal tea made of equal parts hops, lavender flowers,

balm leaves, and primrose, ½ to 1 cup a day taken by mouthfuls as needed, has a natural calming effect.
- A glass of celery juice a day can keep the tranquilizers away.
- Add more B vitamins, niacin, PABA, and magnesium to your daily diet.
- A daily supplement regimen to relieve uptightness is:

Stress B-complex with vitamin C	1 to 3 times daily
Tryptophan	500–667 mg. 1 to 3 times daily
Chelated calcium and magnesium	3 tabs 3 times daily

HIGH BLOOD PRESSURE

- Garlic has blood-pressure-reducing effects. (See sections 126–132 for more information on high blood pressure.)

HEARTBURN

- Try potato juice! Potatoes are a great source of alkaline ingredients which can reduce acidity. Just grate a potato, strain, and drink the juice for natural relief.

STOMACH ACHES

- Because pineapple juice contains an enzyme that helps digest food, drinking a glass of this delicious juice about an hour after you eat can relieve stomach pain.

PALPITATIONS/TACHYCARDIA (RAPID HEARTBEAT)

- Go for rosemary! It's a terrific herb for a variety of ailments—and adds zest to salads, too. Chop some into your daily salads, add to sandwiches and soups.
- Before resorting to other drugs, try Dr. N. G. Hunt's technique of plunging your face into a basin of cool (*not ice cold*) water for about 20 seconds. It causes an almost

immediate reduction in heart rate. (If you have existing heart problems, check with your doctor before trying this method.)

MUSCLE CRAMPS

- Vitamin E (dry) 200–400 IU 3 times daily
- Chelated calcium and magnesium 3 tabs 3 times daily
- Niacin 100 mg. 3 times daily (can cause flushing, redness, and tingling)

NIGHTMARES

- A nice warm cup of camomile tea has often proved to be a good preventive.

SORE THROAT

- Sage soothes a savage throat! Mix ½ oz. of fresh sage leaves with the juice of a lemon or lime. Put the mixture into a quart of boiling water (removed from heat), sweeten to taste with honey, and strain. Drink hot.

IMPOTENCE/DECREASED SEXUAL INTEREST

- Sarsaparilla tea has been used as a sexual stimulant throughout the centuries by the Indians of Mexico. (The sarsaparilla plant has chemical substances with testosterone, progesterone, and cortisol activity, which may account for the plant's usefulness in sexual stimulation.)

WATER RETENTION

- Vitamin B_6, 50 mg. taken 3 times daily is recommended.

MEMORY LOSS

- A good vitamin regimen for this is:

L-glutamine	500 mg. 3 times daily
Vitamin B-complex	50 mg. A.M. and P.M.
Choline	500 mg. 2 times daily

FATIGUE

- This is one of the most common side effects of all medications and one that responds best to a supplement regimen:

Vitamin B complex (time-release)	100 mg. 2 times daily
High potency multiple vitamin & mineral	A.M. & P.M.
Vitamin B_{12}	2,000 mcg. A.M. & P.M.
Vitamin C	1,000 mcg. A.M. & P.M.
Vitamin B_{15}	50 mg. after largest meal of the day

55. Quick reference list of foods that are best sources of vitamins and minerals

VITAMIN	*BEST NATURAL SOURCES*
Vitamin A	fish liver oil, liver, carrots, green and yellow vegetables, eggs, milk and dairy products, margarine, yellow fruits
Vitamin B_1 (thiamine)	dried yeast, rice husks, whole wheat, oatmeal, peanuts, pork, most vegetables, bran, milk
Vitamin B_2 (riboflavin)	milk, liver, kidney, yeast, cheese, leafy green vegetables, fish, eggs
Vitamin B_6 (pyridoxine)	brewer's yeast, wheat bran, wheat germ, liver, kidney, heart, cantaloupe, cabbage, blackstrap molasses, milk, eggs, beef
Vitamin B_{12} (cobalamin)	liver, beef, pork, eggs, milk, cheese, kidney
Vitamin B_{13} (orotic acid)	root vegetables, whey, the liquid portion of soured or curdled milk

VITAMIN	*BEST NATURAL SOURCES*
Vitamin B_{15} (pangamic acid)	brewer's yeast, whole brown rice, whole grains, pumpkin seeds, sesame seeds
Vitamin B_{17} (laetrile)	a small amount of laetrile is found in the whole kernels of apricots, apples, cherries, peaches, plums, and nectarines
Biotin (coenzyme R or vitamin H)	nuts, fruits, brewer's yeast, beef liver, egg yolk, milk, kidney, unpolished rice
Vitamin C (ascorbic acid)	citrus fruits, berries, green and leafy vegetables, tomatoes, cauliflower, potatoes, sweet potatoes
Calcium Pantothenate (Pantothenic acid, Panthenol, vitamin B_5)	meat, whole grains, wheat germ, bran, kidney, liver, heart, green vegetables, brewer's yeast, nuts, chicken, crude molasses
Choline	egg yolk, brain, heart, green leafy vegetables, yeast, liver, wheat germ (and, in small amounts, in lecithin)
Vitamin D (calciferol, viosterol, ergosterol)	fish liver oils, sardines, herring, salmon, tuna, milk and dairy products
Vitamin E (tocopherol)	wheat germ, soybeans, vegetable oils, broccoli, brussels sprouts, leafy greens, spinach, enriched flour, whole wheat, whole grain cereals, eggs

VITAMIN	BEST NATURAL SOURCES
Vitamin F (unsaturated fatty acids—linoleic, linolenic, & arachidonic)	vegetable oils—wheat germ, linseed, sunflower, safflower, soybean, & peanut—peanuts, sunflower seeds, walnuts, pecans, almonds, avocados
Folic acid (folacin)	deep-green leafy vegetables, carrots, tortula yeast, liver, egg yolk, cantaloupe, apricots, pumpkins, avocados, beans, whole wheat & dark rye flour
Inositol	liver, brewer's yeast, dried lima beans, beef brains and heart, cantaloupe, grapefruit, raisins, wheat germ, unrefined molasses, peanuts, cabbage
Vitamin K (menadione)	yogurt, alfalfa, egg yolk, safflower oil, soybean oil, fish liver oils, kelp, leafy green vegetables
Niacin (nicotinic acid, niacinamide, nicotinamide)	liver, lean meat, whole wheat products, brewer's yeast, kidney, wheat germ, fish, eggs, roasted peanuts, the white meat of poultry, avocados, dates, figs, prunes
Vitamin P (C complex, citrus bioflavonoids, rutin, hesperidin)	the white skin and segment part of citrus fruit—lemons, oranges, grapefruit; also in apricots, buckwheat, blackberries, cherries, & rose hips
PABA (para-aminobenzoic acid)	liver, brewer's yeast, kidney, whole grains, rice, bran, wheat germ, & molasses

MINERAL	BEST NATURAL SOURCES
Calcium	milk and milk products, all cheeses, soybeans, sardines, salmon, peanuts, walnuts, sunflower seeds, dried beans, green vegetables
Chlorine	table salt, kelp, olives
Chromium	meat, shellfish, chicken, corn oil, clams, brewer's yeast
Cobalt	milk, kidney, liver, meat, oysters, clams
Copper	dried beans, peas, whole wheat, prunes, calf and beef liver, shrimp and most seafood
Fluorine	seafoods and gelatin
Iodine (iodide)	kelp, vegetables grown in iodine-rich soil, onions, all seafood
Iron	pork liver; beef kidney, heart, and liver; farina, raw clams, dried peaches, red meat, egg yolk, oysters, nuts, beans, asparagus, molasses, oatmeal
Magnesium	figs, lemons, grapefruit, yellow corn, almonds, nuts, seeds, dark green vegetables, apples
Manganese	nuts, green leafy vegetables, peas, beets, egg yolk, whole grain cereals
Molybdenum	dark green leafy vegetables, whole grains, legumes
Phosphorus	fish, poultry, meat, whole grains, eggs, nuts, seeds

MINERAL	BEST NATURAL SOURCES
Potassium	citrus fruits, watercress, all green leafy vegetables, mint leaves, sunflower seeds, bananas, potatoes
Selenium	wheat germ, bran, tuna fish, onions, tomatoes, broccoli
Sodium	salt, shellfish, carrots, beets, artichokes, dried beef, brains, kidney, bacon
Sulfur	lean beef, dried beans, fish, eggs, cabbage
Vanadium	fish
Water	drinking water, juices, fruits and vegetables
Zinc	round steak, lamb chops, pork loin, wheat germ, brewer's yeast, pumpkin seeds, eggs, nonfat dry milk, ground mustard

56. SIDE EFFECT ALERT: Symptoms you don't usually associate with your medication

Very often side effects are confused with symptoms of another illness, because you just can't imagine those symptoms bearing any relationship to the medicine you're taking. A drug to treat nausea, TIGAN (*trimethobenzamide*) for instance, would seem unlikely to be responsible for your back pain—but it could be! The same holds true for other discomforts, such as mouth or eye pains, which frequently send people off to dentists and ophthalmologists for new medications, when the problems are simply the side effects of their present prescriptions. A doctor should always be consulted if any condition is bothersome or causes consternation; but before rushing out for yet another Rx, look over the following list and see if there's any relationship between the way you feel and the drug you're taking.

(NOTE: The list of medications and symptoms is not all-inclusive, and the most common side effects—diarrhea, nausea, constipation, etc.—have been omitted. But if you're not feeling well while getting well, check the specifics on your particular medication in sections 32–52; relief might be just a prescription change away!)

SYMPTOM	ARE YOU TAKING . . .
bloody or black stools	aspirin
	aspirin & codeine
	bromocriptine (PARLODEL)
	diuretics
	anticoagulants
	antiarthritis drugs
	naproxen
	oxycodone & aspirin (PERCODAN)
	antigout medicines
bloody or dark urine	baclofen (LIORESAL)
	anticoagulants
	antihyperlipidemics
	erythromycins
	ethchlorvynol (PLACIDYL)
bluish fingernails or mucous membranes	APC medications
breast soreness	cimetidine (TAGAMET)
	minoxidil (LONITEN)
	spironolactone (ALDACTONE)
changes in menstrual cycle	prochlorperazine & isopropamide (COMBID)
	spironolactone (ALDACTONE)
	any sex hormones
cloudy urine	anthralin (topical)
	APC medications
clumsiness	atropine (ophthalmic)
	barbiturates

SYMPTOM	ARE YOU TAKING . . .
darkening of skin	antithyroid medications estrogen & progestins
decrease in height	heparin
decreased hearing	propoxyphene & APC antiarthritis drugs neomycin oxycodone & aspirin (PERCODAN)
decreased sexual ability	antihyperlipidemics antihypertensives MAO inhibitors
depression/mood changes/mental confusion	adrenocorticoids baclofen (LIORESAL) benzodiazepines beta-blockers antihypertensives estrogens antiarthritis medicines potassium supplements procainamide propoxyphene (DARVON) any sex hormones trimethobenzamide (TIGAN)
difficult or painful urination	appetite suppressants butalbital & APC codeine antispasmodics antiarthritis drugs hydrocodone & pseudoephedrine (TUSSEND) levodopa meperidine (DEMEROL) pentazocine (TALWIN)
drooping eyelids	antihypertensives

SYMPTOM	*ARE YOU TAKING . . .*
eye pain	kaolin, pectin, belladonna alkaloids, and opium (DONNAGEL-PG)
	tricyclic antidepressants
flushing or redness of face	atropine (ophthalmic)
	bethanechol
	butalbital & APC
hallucinations	stimulants
	pargyline (EUTONYL)
	pentazocine (TALWIN)
	procainamide
	tricyclic antidepressants
increased blood pressure	caffeine (APC medicines)
	pseudoephedrine (SUDAFED)
	estrogens & progestins
	amphetamines
	appetite suppressants
increased hair growth	diazoxide (PROGLYCEM)
	phenytoin (DILANTIN)
	spironolactone (ALDACTONE)
increased sensitivity to sunlight	barbiturates
	fertility drugs
	anticonvulsants
	antihypertensives
	nalidixic acid (NEGGRAM)
	oxolinic acid
	estrogens & progestins
	prochlorperazine & isopropamide (COMBID)
	antihistamines
	tetracyclines
	tricyclic antidepressants
increased urination	appetite suppressants
	aspirin & codeine
	butalbital & APC

SYMPTOM	ARE YOU TAKING . . .
	clotrimazole
	cromolyn
	antiarthritis drugs
	hydrocodone & pseudoephedrine (TUSSEND)
	oxycodone & aspirin (PERCODAN)
	pentazocine (TALWIN)
lightening of hair color	antithyroid medications
loss of bladder control	antiglaucoma agents, anticholinergics
nightmares	antihypertensives MAO inhibitors
nighttime urination	antihypertensives
pale stools	erythromycin ethchlorvynol (PLACIDYL)
pink to brownish red discoloration of urine	prochlorperazine & isopropamide (COMBID)
red discoloration of urine on contact with some chlorine bleaches	aminosalicylates
red or purple blisters on hands and feet	ergotamine
ringing or buzzing in the ears	antiarthritis medications
rounding out of the face	adrenocorticoids antidiabetics
seeing halos around lights	adrenocorticoids digitalis medicines oxolinic acid

SYMPTOM	*ARE YOU TAKING . . .*
sore mouth or tongue	cephalosporin griseofulvin meclofenamate (MECLOMEN) diuretics
sores in mouth or throat	benzodiazepines antihyperlipidemics melphalan (ALKERAN) antimetabolites
stiff neck	MAO inhibitors
swallowing difficulty	laxatives
swelling of eyelids, face, lips	barbiturates butalbital & APC
swelling of feet	MAO inhibitors estrogens & progestins
unexplained sore throat/fever	acetaminophen & codeine adrenocorticoids allopurinol amantadine (SYMMETREL) anticoagulants antihistamines antithyroid medications barbiturates benzodiazepines beta-blockers decongestants butalbital & APC chloramphenicol (ophthalmic) chlordiazepoxide & amitriptyline chlorzoxazone & acetaminophen cimetidine (TAGAMET) anticonvulsants diuretics antiarthritis drugs glutethimide (DORIDEN) phenytoin (DILANTIN)

SYMPTOM   *ARE YOU TAKING . . .*

meprobamate
antimetabolites
metronidazole (FLAGYL)
phenothiazines
probenecid
prochloroperazine &
isopropamide (COMBID)
sulfasalazine
antigout medicines
sulfonamides
tricyclic antidepressants
trimethobenzamide (TIGAN)

unusual bruising or   acetaminophen & codeine
  bleeding   allopurinol
antidiabetics
antihistamines
barbiturates
beta-blockers
decongestants
butalbital & APC
chloramphenicol (ophthalmic)
chlordiazepoxide & amitriptyline
chlorzoxazone & acetaminophen
cimetidine (TAGAMET)
anticonvulsants
diuretics
ethchlorvynol (PLACIDYL)
various hypnotics
glutethimide (DORIDEN)
phenytoin (DILANTIN)
meprobamate
antimetabolites
metronidazole (FLAGYL)
miconazole (MONISTAT)
probenecid
prochloroperazine &
isopropamide (COMBID)
sulfasalazine

SYMPTOM	*ARE YOU TAKING . . .*
	antigout medicines
	sulfonamides
	tricyclic antidepressants
	trimethobenzamide (TIGAN)
unusual hair loss	anticoagulants
	antithyroid medications
	antihypertensives
yellowing of eyes and skin	benzodiazepines
	butalbital & APC
	chlordiazepoxide & amitriptyline
	chlorzoxazone & acetaminophen
	antihypertensives
	erythromycins
	estrogens
	diuretics
	phenytoin (DILANTIN)
	MAO inhibitors
	Naproxen
	phenothiazines
	prochloroperazine & isopropamide (COMBID)
	sulfasalazine
	sulfonamides
	tricyclic antidepressants

57. Side effects that can be caused by some natural remedies

ACONITE

Small amounts of a fluid extract of the root of this plant in a cup of warm water have been said to successfully reduce pain and fever, inflammation of the stomach, heart palpitations, and more.

POSSIBLE SIDE EFFECTS

This is one of the few herbs which MUST be used with caution, as an excess can cause heart failure.

COMFREY

Used in teas for alleviating stomach ailments, coughs, diarrhea, arthritis pain, liver and gall bladder conditions.

POSSIBLE SIDE EFFECTS

Can reduce absorption of iron and vitamin B_{12}.

GINSENG

This natural stimulant of both mental and physical energy which has been used for centuries by the Chinese for a variety of ailments including impotence, anemia, arthritis, indigestion, poor circulation, fatigue, and more, can have side effects. It should be noted, though, that not all commercially available products contain the active ingredient of the whole ginseng root in the same proportions—and some contain no detectably active ingredients. Also, be sure to read labels, because there are still other commercial ginseng products that may contain *phenylbutazone* and *aminopyrine*, which have their own side effects.

POSSIBLE SIDE EFFECTS

Hypertension, skin eruptions, nervousness, diarrhea, water retention, breast pain, and, since it can affect blood sugar levels, it might cause problems for diabetics.

LICORICE

Used as a restorer of membrane and tissue function, a hormone balancer, an intestinal secretion stimulant, a respiratory stimulant, and a laxative.

POSSIBLE SIDE EFFECTS

Cardiac arrhythmias, high blood pressure. (American manufactured licorice, the sort used in candy, is a synthetic flavoring and doesn't have these potential side effects—or the benefits.)

PENNYROYAL

Used as an inhalant in treating colds (often called "lung

mint"), it is also used as a tea for curing headaches, menstrual cramps, and pain.

POSSIBLE SIDE EFFECTS

It can induce abortion and should therefore NEVER be used during pregnancy.

MY ADVICE

As a rule, few medical problems occur from ingesting herbal remedies, but you should be aware that the potential for an allergic or toxic response is always there. If you are now taking any drugs, or have any medical problems, it's wise to consult a nutritionally-oriented physician who's aware of herb-drug interactions (substances containing calcium, magnesium, and iron, for instance, can inactivate *tetracycline* drugs) as well as other potentially dangerous side effects.

58. Watch out for the heat!

Heat stroke, which occurs when the body's temperature rises to 105° F (40.5° C) or above, can become a deadly side effect of many commonly prescribed medicines. Before engaging in any strenuous exercise or planning a holiday in the tropics (or even a day at the beach), check with your physician if you are taking any of the following medications:

DRUGS THAT CAN INCREASE YOUR CHANCES OF HEAT STROKE

Anticholinergics containing *atropine*
Antihistamines
COGENTIN (*benztropine mesylate*)
INDERAL (*propanalol*)
HISTORAL, PLEXONAL, UROGESIC (*scopolamine, scopolamine hydrobromide*)
THORAZINE, PROMAPAR, SONAZINE (*chlorpromazine*)
Tricyclic antidepressants (*amitriptyline, desipramine, imipramine, nortriptyline*, and *protriptyline*)

MAO inhibitors (*isocarboxazid, phenelzine, tranylcypromine*)
Inhalational anesthetics (*ether, halothane, nitrous oxide*)
DORIDEN (*glutethimide*)
Any amphetamines
Diuretics

59. Hot tips on your medicines

- Hot weather can speed up chemical reactions in your body and alter the way a drug takes effect—or *doesn't* take effect! (Heat can often cause the body to detoxify and excrete a drug more quickly.)
- Anticoagulants become *more* effective if your body temperature is up.
- A small 2° rise in body temperature can make *digitalis* 10 to 15 percent more toxic.
- CHLOROMYCETIN (*chloramphenicol*) becomes less effective as a topical ointment as temperature rises (and if it's really hot, the medication can cause bacteria to grow faster).
- Sleeping pills change effectiveness according to room temperatures—some become more potent while others become less so.
- Topical *penicillin* and *tetracycline* ointments become more effective in the heat.
- Diet pills containing amphetamines and strenuous exercise can be a lethal combination in very hot weather.
- Hot weather can work with your antihypertensive medication and lower your blood pressure *too* much.
- Any OTC decongestant can affect your body's circulation and should therefore be used cautiously in hot weather.
- Caffeine is a drug and a vasoconstrictor, which means that it should be ingested sparingly in hot weather. (One cola might be refreshing, but a child who drinks three or four while playing at the beach could be in real physical danger.)

60. Any questions about Chapter VII?

I have hypoglycemia and was told not to drink beverages containing caffeine, so I've switched to herb teas. But are there any herb teas that I shouldn't drink?

As a matter of fact, there are. Certain plants have hypoglycemic properties and should be avoided. Among them are: Burdock, Black Cohosh, Coriander, Cranesbill, Dandelion, Fenugreek, Ginseng, Goldenseal, Mugwort, Periwinkle, Solomon's Seal, Sumac, and Snakeroot.

Ever since I began taking the Pill, I've noticed that I have major mood swings. I mean, I go from feeling really depressed to floating on a cloud. Is this all in my mind—or is there some connection with the Pill?

More than likely it's the hormones in the Pill that are causing your depression-to-euphoria jumps. Other drugs, such as the adrenocorticoid *prednisone* (DELTASONE, METICORTEN, ORASONE, STERAPRED) can cause similar mood swings.

I live in Florida and am on a daily regimen of antidepressant drugs (ELAVIL). I enjoy exercise, but don't want to run the risk of heat stroke. What would you suggest?

First, I'd suggest that you discuss the matter with your physician, who is more acquainted with your general physical condition. If you're in good general health, I'd advise that you find yourself an air-conditioned gym and just not overdo things. Avoid tight-fitting dark clothing, and be sure to drink enough liquids to avoid dehydration. If you're overweight, check with your doctor on the right diet for you. DON'T resort to diet pills—they'll only increase your heat-stroke risk.

Part Three

MEALS AND MEDICINES

Chapter VIII

Down the Hatch

61. Nutritious quick pick-me-ups compatible with your medications

IF YOU'RE TAKING . . .

PICK-ME-UPS

Antihypertensives *or*
  Diuretics

These low-sodium and
high-potassium treats can
lift spirits while helping you
feel well:

PEANUT SWIRL

Blend 1 cup lowfat milk,
¼ tsp. cinnamon, ¼ cup
unsalted peanut butter,
⅓ tsp. light molasses,
2–4 ice cubes

JUICY-FRUITY

Blend 1 cup cantaloupe,
½ cup orange juice, juice of
½ lemon, and ice

IF YOU'RE TAKING . . .	PICK-ME-UPS
Antibiotics	Because antibiotics deplete vitamin K as well as kill off a great number of good bacteria along with the bad, a delicious and helpful midafternoon snack would be this one:

BANANA-YO FREEZY

Blend ½ banana, ½ cup plain yogurt, dash of cinnamon, and ice.

Antihistamines *or* Decongestants	Vitamin C-rich foods are what you want, and a terrific C booster is this tasty drink:

ORANGE ANGEL

Blend ½ cup orange juice, ¾ cup pineapple juice, ¼ cup nonfat dry milk, ¼ cup blanched almonds, and ½ cup ice.

Antihyperlipidemics	A holiday treat with only 7 milligrams of cholesterol!

UN-EGGNOG

Beat together 1 egg white, 1 cup chilled skim milk, 1 tsp. NutraSweet, a pinch of salt, dash of cinnamon, ¼ tsp. vanilla. Sprinkle with nutmeg and enjoy.

Antispasmodics *or* Anticholinergics	This slick beverage can soothe your tummy, satisfy your sweet tooth, and step up your energy at the same time.

IF YOU'RE TAKING . . .   *PICK-ME-UPS*

SILKY BANAPPLE

Blend ½ large banana, 1
cup apple juice, 1 T protein
powder, and 1 scoop
natural vanilla ice cream.

Appetite
    Suppressants

Try this quickie for
breakfast or a snack. It's
nutritious and only 150
calories! (You can even
freeze it and use it as a
dessert for dinner.)

IO'S AMBROSIA

Blend 1 cup (8 oz.) nonfat
or low-fat milk (or juice),
a flavored low-calorie
protein powder that
contains nutritional yeast,
lecithin, fructose, and 4–6
ice cubes.

Cardiovascular
    drugs

The best way I know to
treat your heart is to give it
enough vitamins B, C, and
E. And this tasty tonic has
them all.

HEART'S DELIGHT

Blend ½ cup orange (or
other fresh citrus fruit)
juice, ½ cup tomato juice,
1 T brewer's yeast powder,
and 5–6 T cold-pressed
wheat germ oil.

Tranquilizers *and*
    Sedatives

A superb drink for fostering
sweet dreams and tranquil
afternoons—while giving you
energy, too—is this simple
calcium-rich mixture:

IF YOU'RE TAKING . . .   *PICK-ME-UPS*

MORPHEUS' MAGIC

> Blend 1–2 bananas
> (depending on size), 1 cup
> low-fat or skim milk, and 2
> T honey.

62. How to stop vitamin thieves

Almost every drug you take takes something from you.
But being forewarned is being forearmed, and being prepared
to arm yourself nutritionally with the right foods and supplements is your best defense against vitamin thieves.

VITAMIN THIEF	*STOLEN NUTRIENTS*	*YOUR DEFENSE*
Alcohol (including alcohol-containing cough syrups, elixirs, and OTC medications such as NYQUIL.)	Vitamins A, B_1, B_2, biotin, choline, niacin, vitamin B_{15}, folic acid, & magnesium	B-complex supple-ment; nutritional yeast, liver, whole brown rice, whole grain cereals, pumpkin and sesame seeds, wheat germ
Ammonium Chloride (e.g. AMBENYL EXPECTORANT, TRIAMINICOL DECONGESTANT COUGH SYRUP, P-V TUSSIN SYRUP)	Vitamin C	Vitamin C: fresh fruits and vegetables
Antacids (e.g. MAALOX, MY-LANTA, GELUSIL, TUMS, ROLAIDS)	B-complex & Vitamin A	B-complex, vitamin A; fish liver oils, yeast, and liver

VITAMIN THIEF	STOLEN NUTRIENTS	YOUR DEFENSE
Anticoagulants (e.g., COUMADIN, DICUMAROL, PANWARFIN)	Vitamins A & K	Vitamin A; fish liver oil, alfalfa, yogurt, kelp, leafy green vegetables*
Antihistamines (e.g. CHLOR-TRIMETON, PYRIBENZAMINE)	Vitamin C	Vitamin C; fresh fruits & vegetables
Aspirin (and remember, APC drugs contain *aspirin*)	Vitamin A, B-complex, C; calcium, potassium	Vitamins A, C; eggs, milk, nutritional yeast, desiccated liver, fresh fruits & vegetables
Barbiturates (e.g. PHENOBARBITAL, SECONAL, NEM-BUTAL, BUTISOL, TUINAL)	Vitamins A, D, folic acid, & C	fish liver oil, vitamins A, D, and folic acid; green leafy vegetables, vitamin C, fresh fruits & vegetables
Caffeine (present in all APC medicines)	B_1, inositol & biotin; potassium, zinc, can also inhibit calcium & iron assimilation	B_1, inositol & biotin or B complex supplement; wheat germ, bran, rice polish, nutritional yeast, blackstrap molasses
Chloramphenicol (CHLORO-MYCETIN)	Vitamin K & niacin	alfalfa, yogurt, kelp, leafy green vegetables; niacin or nicotinic acid, nutritional yeast, desiccated liver

*Important: foods containing high amounts of vitamin K (see section 55) can reverse the blood-thinning action of anticoagulants!

VITAMIN THIEF	STOLEN NUTRIENTS	YOUR DEFENSE
Clofibrate (ATROMID-S)	Vitamin K	alfalfa, yogurt, kelp, leafy green vegetables
Colchicine (COLBENEMID)	B_{12}, A, and potassium	Vitamins B_{12}, A & potassium; liver, beef, pork, fish liver oil, bananas, tomato juice, potatoes, raw sunflower seeds
Diethylstilbestrol (DES)	Vitamin B_6	Vitamin B_6; nutritional yeast, desiccated liver
Diuretics (e.g. DIURIL, HYDRODIURIL, SER-AP-ES, LASIX)	B-complex, potassium, magnesium, & zinc	complete multiple B-complex, multiple mineral; bananas, tomato juice, raw sunflower seeds, apples
Fluorides	Vitamin C	Vitamin C, fresh fruits and vegetables
Glutethimide (DORIDEN)	Folic acid	folic acid; green leafy vegetables
Indomethacin (INDOCIN)	Vitamins B_1 & C	Vitamins B_1 & C; wheat germ, bran, nutritional yeast
Isoniazid (INH, NYDRAZID)	B_6	B_6; nutritional yeast, desiccated liver
Kanamycin (KANTREX)	Vitamins K & B_{12}	alfalfa, yogurt, kelp, leafy green vegetables; liver, beef, pork

VITAMIN THIEF	STOLEN NUTRIENTS	YOUR DEFENSE
Laxatives, lubricant (e.g. castor oil, mineral oil)	Vitamins A, D, E, K, calcium, & phosphorus	Vitamins A, D, & E supplements; kelp, alfalfa, green vegetables, yogurt, kafir, milk, bone meal
Meprednisone (BETAPAR)	Vitamins B_6, C, zinc, & potassium	B_6, zinc, and potassium supplements; nutritional yeast, liver, fresh fruits & vegetables, bananas, tomato juice, oysters, whole wheat
Methotrexate (MEXATE)	Folic acid	folic acid; green leafy vegetables
Nitrofurantoin (e.g. FURADANTIN, MACRODANTIN)	Folic acid	folic acid; green leafy vegetables
Oral contraceptives (e.g. BREVICON, DEMULEN, ENOVID, LO/ OVRAL, NORINYL, OVRAL)	Folic acid, C, B_2, B_6, B_{12}, & E	B-complex, C & E; wheat germ, nutritional yeast, desiccated liver, dairy products, fish, leafy green vegetables
Penicillamine (CUPRIMINE)	Vitamin B_6	B_6, nutritional yeast, desiccated liver
Penicillin (in all its forms)	Vitamins B_6, niacin, & K	B-complex, nutritional yeast, desiccated liver, alfalfa, yogurt, kelp, leafy green vegetables

VITAMIN THIEF	STOLEN NUTRIENTS	YOUR DEFENSE
Phenylbutazone (e.g. AZOLID, BUTAZOLIDIN)	Folic acid	folic acid; green leafy vegetables
Phenytoin (DILANTIN)	Folic acid & vitamin D	folic acid; green leafy vegetables, fish liver oil
Prednisone (e.g. METICORTEN, PREDNISOLONE, ORASONE)	Vitamins B_6, D, C, zinc, & potassium	B complex with C & zinc and potassium supplements; nutritional yeast, desiccated liver, fish liver oils, fresh fruits and vegetables, oysters, whole wheat, bananas, tomato juice, potatoes
Propantheline (PRO-BANTHINE)	Vitamin K	alfalfa, yogurt, kelp, leafy green vegetables
Pyrimethamine (DARAPRIM)	Folic acid	folic acid; green leafy vegetables
Sulfonamides, systemic (e.g. BACTRIM, GANTANOL, GANTRISIN, SEPTRA)	Folic acid, vitamins K & B_2	Vitamin B-complex; leafy green vegetables, liver, nutritional yeast; tongue and other organ meats
Sulfonamides and topical steroids (e.g. AEROSPORIN, CORTISPORIN, NEOSPORIN, POLYSPORIN)	Vitamins K, B_{12} & folic acid	alfalfa, yogurt, kelp, leafy green vegetables; liver, beef, pork; folic acid

VITAMIN THIEF	STOLEN NUTRIENTS	YOUR DEFENSE
Tetracyclines (e.g. ACHROMYCIN-V, SUMYCIN, TETRACYN)	Vitamin K, calcium, magnesium, & iron	alfalfa, yogurt, kelp, green leafy vegetables; milk, grapefruit, almonds, organ meats, asparagus; a multiple mineral supplement
Tobacco	Vitamin C, B_1, and folic acid; calcium & folic acid	Vitamin C; fresh fruits and vegetables; folic acid; milk; multiple mineral with calcium
Trifluoperazine (STELAZINE)	Vitamin B_{12}	Vitamin B_{12}, iron & folic acid; liver, heart, lean meat, green leafy vegetables, nutritional yeast, dairy products
Triamterene (DYRENIUM)	Folic acid	folic acid; green leafy vegetables

63. Optimum nutrition while getting well

Virtually everyone knows that a balanced diet means eating foods from the four basic food groups (milk, meat, fruit/vegetable, and grain) each day—though you couldn't prove it by what most people actually *do* consume on a daily basis.

The three most important things to keep in mind when organizing any meals are:

1. Nutrients work together in teams.
2. One nutrient cannot make up for the shortage of another.
3. Variety in a diet is the best defense against overconsumption or deficiency of any nutrient.

If you're in good health, this is really all you need to know to maintain a good nutritional equilibrium. But if you're on medication, you should learn how to make everything you eat help you toward optimum nutrition.

Take proteins, for instance. These are used by your body to build new tissue and repair damaged cells. They're also used to make hormones and enzymes, keep the acid-alkaline blood content balanced, and eliminate the garbage, among other things.

As protein is digested, it is broken down into smaller compounds called amino acids. When these amino acids reach the cells in your body, they're formed into protein again. It's a wonderful cycle.

Though the same twenty-two amino acids form all proteins (and there are thousands of them), they each perform a different function in a different area of the body.

Proteins can be divided into two classes—complete and incomplete. Complete protein provides the proper balance of necessary amino acids. Incomplete protein lacks certain essential amino acids and is not used efficiently when eaten alone. However, when small amounts of complete (animal source) protein are combined with incomplete protein, the combination can give you better nutrition than either one alone!

> By combining these complete proteins—cheese, eggs, fish, meat, milk, poultry—with these incomplete proteins—bread, cereal, dried beans, fruits, pasta, nuts, rice and vegetables—you get more nutritive value than either could provide alone!

Carbohydrates are also important. They provide the energy needed to assist in the digestion and assimilation of all the foods you eat.

Carbohydrates break down inside cells to release energy. In fact, the main source of the brain's energy is the sugar glucose, which comes primarily from starch in the diet. Of course if the energy isn't needed, the carbohydrates are stored in the liver as glycogen for later use, and, unfortunately, since there's a limit to what the liver can handle, the excess is converted into body fat. And as if this weren't bad enough, the excess can also cause a vitamin B deficiency because your B vitamins will be called from other metabolic needs to burn up the unnecessary carbohydrates.

Just keep in mind that there are helpful carbohydrates and harmful carbohydrates. The helpful ones are: whole grains (wheat, rye, barley), whole-grain cereals, whole-grain breads, brown rice, vegetables, fresh vegetable juices, fresh fruit juices, and fruits.

The harmful carbohydrates are: refined white sugar, potato chips, snack pies, cakes and cookies, carbonated soft drinks, chewing gum, chocolate and other candies.

And don't forget about fats either. They're as necessary as protein and carbohydrates, though not in the same amounts. (They have twice as many calories per gram as proteins or carbohydrates.)

The reason why fats are important in a proper diet is because they aid in hormone development, promote healthy blood vessels, ensure proper structure of all cells (especially those essential for memory and digestion), assist in controlling the functions of key glands and important chemical reactions which enable enzymes to work and provide the necessary elements for absorption of oil-soluble vitamins such as vitamins A, D, E, and K, as well as other nutrients.

But though all fats contain the same chemical elements of glycerol and fatty acids, they are not the same because the glycerol and fatty acids are not present in the same amounts.

Saturated fat is the type that's usually solid when at room temperature. This is found in meats (coconut, too) and can increase the amount of cholesterol in the blood.

Unsaturated fat (monounsaturated or polyunsaturated) is usually liquid and comes primarily from vegetable sources. Unsaturated fats don't raise cholesterol levels and polyunsaturated fats actually lower them!

64. Keeping energy up while taking medicine

Unless contraindicated by your particular medical problem or medication, I recommend that you step up your protein consumption at every meal. A simple way to do this is with a good pep-up protein drink.

PROTEIN POWERHOUSE

2 tbsp. protein powder	1 tbsp. nutritional yeast
1 tbsp. lecithin powder	1 tbsp. safflower oil (optional)
2 tbsp. acidophilus liquid	

Blend with milk, water, or juice for 1 minute.

As for supplements, the following is the best high-energy regimen I know:

WITH BREAKFAST

High-potency multiple vitamin with chelated minerals (time release preferred)
Stress B complex with C
Vitamin E (200–400 IU)
High-potency multiple chelated mineral
Acidophilus, 3 capsules or 2 tbsp. liquid
Lecithin granules, 1 tbsp. (or 3 1,200 mg. capsules)

WITH LUNCH

Calcium and magnesium tablets (3)
Stress B-complex with C
Vitamin E (200–400 IU)
Acidophilus, 3 capsules or 2 tbsp. liquid
(Optional: Vitamin B_{12}, liver tablets, digestive enzymes)

WITH DINNER

Stress B-complex with C
Vitamin E (200–400 IU)
Acidophilus, 3 capsules or 2 tbsp. liquid
Lecithin granules, 1 tbsp. or 3 1,200 mg. capsules
(Optional: digestive enzymes)

65. Any questions about Chapter VIII?

When I'm on medication and don't feel well enough to eat, what vitamins can I take to ensure a balanced diet?

I think you're under the misapprehension that vitamins are substitutes for food. Well, they're not. Nor are they substitutes for protein, other nutrients, or even for each other. You can't stop eating, take vitamins, and expect to be healthy. If you're unable to eat solids, at least make sure that you're getting enough nutritious liquids (milk, juices, broths, etc.). The Protein Powerhouse drink mentioned in section 64, along with the supplement regimens listed below it, should tide you over until your appetite returns.

Part Four

IT TAKES ALL KINDS

Chapter IX

Women's Drugs

66. The Pill: Pro and Con

PRO

- It's one of the most effective and convenient reversible contraceptives available.
- It can cure severe menstrual distress by eliminating menstruation. (Pills that contain progestin and estrogen—"combination type"—prevent ovulation and menstruation. What occurs monthly is actually "withdrawal bleeding," which is commonly referred to as menstruation.)
- According to a Boston University School of Medicine study, oral combination-type contraceptives may have a protective effect against cancer of the uterus.

CON

- It increases your risk of developing blood clots.
- You're three to six times as susceptible to heart attacks.
- It doubles your risk of suffering a stroke, more than doubles it if you're a smoker (see section 49).
- It increases your risk of gall bladder disease.

- It may cause liver tumors and/or cancer of the liver.
- Six percent of pill users get pregnant during the first year due to a combination of user failure and the body's requisite first cycle period of adjustment.
- Women who become pregnant while taking the pill run the risk of having a child with birth defects.
- It can decrease your glucose tolerance, worsening symptoms of hypoglycemia (dizziness, fatigue, mental disturbance).
- It may cause users to develop high blood pressure.
- Sequential pills (which contain estrogen and progestin in a sequence more like a natural cycle) may increase the risk of cancer of the endometrium.

> Pill users are more susceptible to VD.

- Early-stage cancer of the cervix has been shown to be higher in pill users.
- Progestin-only pills, which are less likely to cause high blood pressure and clots than pills that also contain estrogen, are also less likely to prevent conception.
- The acid-alkaline balance of the vagina is altered by the Pill, making users more susceptible to a variety of vaginal infections and venereal disease.
- After going off the Pill, women who've had a history of menstrual irregularity might not be able to ovulate again.
- Skin discolorations caused by the Pill are generally not reversible.
- Many eye problems (such as double vision, contact lens intolerance, swelling of the eye membranes, inflammation of the cornea, and more) have been linked to the Pill.
- Users with a history of benign breast disease have a greater chance of contracting breast cancer.
- The Pill can decrease your sex drive.
- It depletes you of vitamins C, B_6, B_{12}, folic acid, magnesium, and zinc.

- One out of every three pill users shows depressive personality changes.
- It can cause or exacerbate colitis.
- Pain, joint-swelling, and other arthritis-type symptoms can be a side effect of the Pill.

67. Recipes for Pill users

SUPER C FRUIT COCKTAIL

Cut up sections of fresh oranges, grapefruit, bananas, cantaloupe, honeydew, peaches, and tangerines. Mix in bowl. Trickle some honey and wheat germ over fruit, then slice strawberries and layer across the top. Chill and serve. (Great as an appetizer, dessert, or snack.)

BEAUTIFUL B_6 SALMON-AVOCADO MOUSSE

1 cup cold water
1 tbsp. aspartame (Equal, NutraSweet)
2 tbsp. fresh lemon juice
1 tbsp. white wine vinegar
2½ tbsp. grated onion
2 tbsp. horseradish
1 1-pound can red salmon
½ cup mayonnaise
1 package unflavored gelatin

Soften the gelatin in cold water. Stir over low heat until completely dissolved. Add aspartame, lemon juice, vinegar, onion, and horseradish. Chill.

When mixture is almost set, fold in salmon and mayonnaise. Spoon into mold and chill until firm.

AVOCADO DRESSING

Peel and mash 1 large avocado and blend with ½ cup sour cream. Serve with mousse.

FULL-OF-FOLIC-ACID SALAD*

Use plenty of fresh dark leafy greens (including watercress, parsley, chicory, and beet greens), sprinkle with chopped walnuts, slivered almonds, and if desired some grated cheddar cheese.

---

*And there's magnesium in there, too!

MAGIC MINT DRESSING

1 cup salad oil	¼ tsp. basil
1 cup red wine vinegar	¼ tsp. fresh ground pepper
1 clove garlic (split)	¼ tsp. chopped fresh mint

Put all ingredients in jar and refrigerate for 24 hours. Remove garlic and shake vigorously before serving.

REMEMBER: If you're on the Pill, you're getting ripped off nutritionally, so pay attention to your diet and eat foods that count! If you don't feel that you are, here are some supplement suggestions:

•High potency multiple vitamin with chelated minerals (time-release)	A.M. & P.M.
•Vitamin C	1,000 mg. A.M. & P.M.
•Zinc (chelated)	50 mg. 1 to 3 times daily
•Folic acid	400 mcg. 1 to 3 times daily
•Vitamin B_{12}	2,000 mcg. A.M.
•Vitamin B_6	50 mg. 1 to 3 times daily

68. Pregnant and nursing mothers' guide to medicines

No drug—whether it's OTC or prescription, alcohol, nicotine, or caffeine—should be considered safe during pregnancy! (Most drugs can cross the placenta and thus affect fetus as well as mother.) And when you consider that the major stages in an embryo's development occur during the first few weeks of life, before most women even *know* that they're pregnant, it's wise, if you're even *contemplating* motherhood, to think twice and check with a physician before taking *any* medicine.

- Overuse of *aspirin* or salicylate analgesics such as ANACIN, BUFFERIN, ALKA-SELTZER, and so on, especially in the third trimester, may prolong pregnancy or labor, and can cause severe bleeding in both mother and newborn before, during, and after delivery.
- When antacids, such as ROLAIDS, MAALOX, MILK OF MAGNESIA, CAMALOX, and others, are taken for

prolonged periods, or in high doses, they may cause muscle problems in the fetus. (Sodium antacids can cause pregnant women to retain too much water.)

- Some anticough medicines, such as *terpin hydrate* products, contain large amounts of alcohol, which can cause birth defects, so be aware of how much more alcohol you're adding to your daily intake.
- Regular use of antidiarrheals containing *paregoric* may lead to drug dependency in newborns and cause withdrawal symptoms. (If taken just prior to delivery, these medications can cause breathing problems in newborns.)
- Topical hydrocortisone products used to treat hemorrhoids (ANUSOL-HC) can, if used in large amounts or for prolonged periods of time, be absorbed through the skin and cause birth defects.
- Some prescription antinausea preparations containing *doxylamine* with *pyridoxine* might cause birth defects.
- Taking *phenothiazine* products (THORAZINE, COMPAZINE, PHENERGAN) can cause jaundice and muscle tremors in newborns.
- *Tetracyclines* are not recommended for use in the last half of pregnancy, because they may cause discoloration of forming teeth in newborns as well as retard the growth of teeth and bones in infants.
- *Pseudoephedrine* decongestants (SUDAFED) may cause a reduction in size and rate of bone formation in the fetus.
- Amphetamine appetite suppressants such as DEXEDRINE may increase chances of birth defects.
- Routine use of diuretics (HYGROTON, HYDRO-DIURIL, LASIX) is dangerous to mother and fetus and may cause liver and/or blood disorders in newborns.
- Bulk-forming laxatives (SERUTAN, EFFERSYLLIUM) which contain large amounts of sodium or sugar may increase your blood pressure or cause water retention.
- Saline laxatives (EPSOM SALTS, CITRATE OF MAGNESIA, PHOSPHO-SODA) containing magnesium or potassium should be avoided if your kidney functions are not normal; those containing sodium should be avoided if you tend to retain water.
- Repeated use of mineral oil as a laxative can decrease

absorption of foods, vitamins, and oral medications, as well as cause blood disorders in newborns.
- Castor oil may cause contractions in the womb.
- *Quinine,* which can be purchased OTC, may cause birth defects and stimulate premature labor.
- Tranquilizers and sedatives such as SECONAL, PHE-NOBARBITAL, LIBRIUM, VALIUM, DALMANE, and others may increase the chance of birth defects. These drugs may also cause dependency and withdrawal symptoms in newborns. (Used late in pregnancy or during labor, they may cause breathing problems in newborns.)

DRUGS THAT MAY HARM A NURSING BABY

If you're a nursing mother, consult your doctor before taking any medication. Many drugs can enter breast milk—and what's good for you is not necessarily good for your child.

DRUG	CATEGORY
atropine (ATROPISOL)	ophthalmological
barbiturates	sedative/tranquilizer
belladonna alkaloids and barbiturates (drugs containing *atropine, hyoscyamine, scopolamine, butabarbital, pentobarbital, phenobarbital* or *amobarbital*)	antispasmodic/anticholinergic
benzodiazepines	tranquilizer/sedative
cascara sagrada	stimulant laxative
chloramphenicol (CHLOROMYCETIN)	antibiotic
corticosteroids	anti-inflammatory
cyclophosphamide (CYTOXAN)	antineoplastic
danthron (DORBANE, MODANE)	stimulant laxative

DRUG	CATEGORY
dicumarol	anticoagulant
ergotamine (ERGOMAR, ERGOSTAT)	antimigraine
estrogens	hormone
isoniazid (INH, NYDRAZID)	tuberculosis
lithium carbonate	antidepressant
meprobamate (EQUANIL, MILTOWN)	tranquilizer/sedative
methotrexate (MEXATE)	antineoplastic
metronidazole (FLAGYL)	anti-infective
nalidixic acid (NEGGRAM)	urinary antibacterial
oral contraceptives	hormone
penicillin G sodium	antibiotic
phenolphthalein (EX-LAX, FEEN-A-MINT)	stimulant laxative
phenytoin (DILANTIN)	anticonvulsant
potassium iodide (PIMA)	expectorant
primodone (MYSOLINE)	anticonvulsant
streptomycin	antibiotic
sulfisoxazole (GANTRISIN)	urinary antibacterial
tetracycline	antibiotic
thiazides (see section 40)	diuretic
warfarin (COUMADIN, PANWARFARIN)	anticoagulant

Note: The fact that your particular medication does not appear on the above list should in no way be construed that it is harmless to your nursing infant. *Always* consult your doctor before taking a medicine if you are breast feeding!)

69. What you should know about ERT (Estrogen Replacement Therapy)

When a woman reaches menopause, somewhere around the age of 50, there is a decline in her production of estrogen. Because of this, many doctors prescribe estrogen to treat and allegedly prevent aging and its attendant discomforts.

> There is NO medical evidence to support the belief that estrogens will keep you young.

Estrogens such as TACE (*chlorotrianisene*), DES (*diethylstilbestrol*), PREMARIN (*conjugated estrogens*), OGEN (*estropipate*), and ESTINYL (*ethinyl estradiol*) are effective in treating moderate to severe *vasomotor* symptoms, such as hot flashes, associated with menopause, or the postoperative effects of ovary removal, such as the atrophying or drying of vaginal mucous membranes. They are only "probably" effective in treating estrogen deficiency-induced osteoporosis, and then only when used with other therapeutic measures. But there is NO medical evidence to support the belief that estrogens will prevent the appearance of wrinkles, the aging of skin, or, in effect, keep you young. Nor, despite advertising claims to the contrary, is there any evidence that estrogens are effective for treating nervous symptoms and depression associated with menopause. *But there IS evidence that estrogens can increase the risk of endometrial cancer!*

Before rushing out for an estrogen prescription, keep these facts in mind:

- No more than 10 to 20 percent of women going through menopause suffer extreme discomfort.
- The hormonal imbalance that occurs at menopause is temporary, much like the changes which occur at puberty.
- Hot flashes usually last no more than two years, and, as a general rule, are *not* incapacitating.
- Women who've been on estrogen therapy often find that it only delays hot flashes, which then seem to develop when the drug is discontinued.

70. Making your way through menopause naturally

GINSENG

The Chinese have been using ginseng for a variety of ailments for nearly five thousand years, and many women have found it helpful in alleviating the distress of hot flashes. Available as tea, liquid concentrate, or as ginseng root in a bottle, Siberian or Korean ginseng can also be purchased in easy-to-take capsule form.

I'd recommend 500 mg. taken on an empty stomach A.M. and P.M. (Vitamin C has been said to neutralize part of ginseng's value; but if you take a time-release C supplement, it will make counteraction less likely.)

VITAMIN E (with selenium)

Both vitamin E and selenium are antioxidants, slowing down aging and hardening of tissues through oxidation. They are also synergistic, which means that the two together are more effective than the sum of the equal parts. For relief of menopausal distress, I'd suggest starting with 200 mg. and increasing to 400 mg. (mixed tocopherols preferred) 1 to 3 times daily.

L–TRYPTOPHAN

A natural sedative and antidepressant, L-Tryptophan can be quite helpful during menopause. Found in warm milk and turkey, it's also available in supplement form. I'd suggest 3 tryptophan tablets ½ hour before bedtime taken with water or juice (no protein).

CALCIUM AND MAGNESIUM

Calcium and magnesium, more of nature's tranquilizers, can help treat osteoporosis (the porous bone disease caused by demineralization due to lack of estrogen), backache, and muscle cramps that often cause sleeplessness during menopause.

I'd suggest 1 chelated calcium and magnesium tablet 3 times daily.

HERB TEAS

Many herb teas have a soothing and mood-elevating effect, which can be particularly helpful during this period. Camomile (and camomile-based) tea can help turn grizzly-bear moods into teddy-bear ones. Teas containing passion flower (*passiflora*) are also helpful and work as effective sleeping aids.

Valerian is another calming herb—and a potent one. If using the root to make tea, add only half a teaspoon to a cup of boiling water, then let it cool. Drink only one cup a day—and no more than a mouthful at a time.

EXERCISE

Repeated studies have shown that there is a definite relationship between exercise and general well-being. Exercise tones up the circulatory system, gives you more vitality, and can even prevent bone loss as well as strengthen the ligaments between bones, lowering the possibility of fractures, which occur so easily in older people.

Walking briskly is terrific exercise, especially if you're not used to doing any sort of formal workout. (*Always check with your doctor, though, before beginning any sort of exercise regimen.*) Swimming and bike-riding are also effective. I've found that jumping rope is great for general toning up (and you don't have to worry about the weather outside to do it)!

The important thing to remember is that regular exercise—fifteen minutes a day or a half-hour three times a week—is better than one exhausting workout a month . . . and almost any exercise is better than none!

71. Any questions about Chapter IX?

Are there any drugs that can interact with the Pill and cause it to become ineffective as a contraceptive?

As a matter of fact, quite a few drugs may undermine the contraceptive action of the Pill. Among them are antihistamines; barbiturates such as AMYTAL, NEMBUTAL, *phenobarbital,* and SECONAL; BUTAZOLIDIN, DILANTIN, EQUANIL, MILTOWN, RIFADIN, and RIMACTANE. If you plan to rely on the Pill, be sure to discuss *all* your other medications with your physician.

Can having a couple of highballs a night really harm my unborn baby?

Yes, especially in the early months of pregnancy. Alcohol consumption levels as low as 2 standard shots of hard liquor twice a week have produced sizable and significant increases in spontaneous abortions.

Do you know any natural ways to alleviate premenstrual syndrome?

Diet modification is the best way to combat PMS (premenstrual syndrome). For the week before and during your menstrual period:

- Avoid or minimize your intake of salt (see section 130) to lessen water retention.
- Avoid licorice, which can stimulate the production of aldosterone and cause retention of sodium and water.
- Keep away from cold foods and beverages, which can adversely affect abdominal circulation and contribute to cramping.
- Don't drink astringent black teas; the tannin can bind important minerals and inhibit their absorption. (Adding milk to tea takes out some tannin, but not all.)
- Stay away from alcoholic beverages. (Alcohol can lower magnesium levels, affect blood sugar, and adversely affect liver function, which in turn can aggravate PMS symptoms.)
- Minimize your intake of spinach, beet greens, and other oxalate-containing vegetables which can inhibit the assimilation of important minerals.
- Increase your consumption of naturally diuretic foods, such as strawberries, watermelon (seeds, too), artichokes, asparagus, parsley, and watercress.
- Eat more potassium rich foods (see section 55).

Also, a supplement regimen that can help is:

•High potency multiple   A.M. and P.M.
vitamin with chelated minerals

•Vitamin B$_6$	50–300 mg. daily (work up from 50 mg. gradually)
•Vitamin E	100–600 IU daily
•Vitamin C	1,000 mg. daily
•Pantothenic acid	1,000 mg. daily
•Evening Primrose Oil capsules or tablets	1–3 times daily (for 2 to 3 months)

Evening Primrose Oil has been found by many women to reduce physical discomfort as well as mood swings; vitamin E helps reduce premenstrual breast tenderness. And keep in mind, too, that exercise which stimulates the circulation can also help. A brisk half-hour walk twice a day can ease anxiety and benefit you physically as well.

Would there be any problem with my taking VALIUM while I'm on the Pill?

There could be a big one. Recent studies have shown that even low dose birth control pills seem to inhibit the metabolism of VALIUM, meaning that if you take both drugs you run a greater risk of incurring VALIUM toxicity.

Chapter X

Children's Medicines

72. Special cautions when mixing kids and medicines

When prescribed and taken correctly, medicines can cure a variety of children's illnesses that could not be combatted any other way. But far too often, unfortunately, medicines are prescribed for kids (by parents as well as doctors) needlessly, without sufficient instructions for their proper administration, and with no regard for the nutritional toll they can take on a growing youngster.

The following is a list of basic cautions, nutritional precautions, and facts you should know about the medicines you give your children. (For information on adjusting dosages for kids, see section 18, and for special tips on giving medicines, see section 19.)

ASPIRIN

Included in this category are all products containing *aspirin* (*salicylates*), including prescription and over-the-counter APC (*aspirin, phenacetin,* and *caffeine*) drugs such as EMPIRIN, NORGESIC, ASPERGUM, ALKA-SELTZER, CONGESPIRIN, and others.)

- Children below the age of 12 should not take this medicine for more than 5 consecutive days.
- If your child has had *aspirin* prescribed for postoperative oral surgery or tonsil removal, be sure that he or she swallows and does not chew the *aspirin* during this period.
- Taking this medicine with food or milk will lessen the child's chances of stomach upset.
- Never place *aspirin* tablets directly on a tooth or gum surface—they can cause a burn.
- *Aspirin* is a blood thinner and should not be given to a child for 5 days before any surgery (including dental) unless the doctor says so.
  half
- If your child is taking buffered *aspirin* (or *carbaspirin*) for fever and a *tetracycline* antibiotic for infection, the two medicines should not be taken within 1 hour of each other, as the former can inhibit the absorption of the latter.
- Check labels of all OTC medications to make sure that they don't also contain *aspirin* or *phenacetin,* which could lead to overdose.
- *Aspirin* can triple your child's excretion of vitamin C and deplete essential vitamin B_1 (thiamine) and folic acid. (Be sure to replace these nutrients by lacing your child's diet with ample amounts of citrus fruits and juices, nutritional yeast, leafy green vegetables, and other foods high in B vitamins. A good vitamin B-complex with C would be in order.)
- *Aspirin* (and other *salicylates*) have recently been linked to Reye's syndrome (RS) in children. (RS occurs mostly in children under 16 who are recovering from viral infections, particularly influenza and chicken pox. Symptoms are vomiting and lethargy, which may progress to delirium, coma, and even death.) Though all the evidence is not yet in, my advice is: "When in doubt, do without." In other words, if your child has fever with the flu or chicken pox, find another antipyretic.

ACETAMINOPHEN
(TYLENOL, DATRIL, NEBS, TEMPRA, VALADOL)

- Taking this medicine for more than 5 days in a row is not recommended for children under the age of 12.
- Carbohydrates, such as crackers or jellies, can slow the medicine's absorption rate and increase the time it takes to be effective.
- Overdoses of this medicine in children are common, so administer with care.

PENICILLIN and AMPICILLIN
(PENICILLIN G, PEN-VEE K, V-CILLIN K, COMPOCILLIN-V, PENTIDS, AMCILL, POLYCILLIN, OMNIPEN, PENSORB, PRINCIPEN)

- These drugs work best when given to your child on an empty stomach (at least 30 minutes before he or she eats).
- Taking any of these drugs with soft drinks or citrus juices decreases their antibacterial action.
- These antibiotics rob your child of potassium, which should be replaced: make sure the youngster's diet includes bananas, potatoes (with skin), plenty of citrus fruits, tomatoes, sunflower seeds, and yogurt.
- If your child is diabetic, be aware that *ampicillin, hetacillin* (which breaks down to *ampicillin* in the body), and *penicillin G* may cause inaccurate results on some urine sugar tests.
- Don't be distressed by a dark or discolored tongue; it's due to the medicine and will go away.
- A good supplement program for any child on these medications would be a children's multiple-vitamin and mineral, vitamin C (500–1,000 mg.), a stress B complex, and zinc (15 mg.).
- For more information on antibiotics, see section 33.

TETRACYCLINES
(all of them—and the "-mycins")

- These medications should not be given to your child

with milk, dairy products, or food high in iron; they inhibit absorption (see section 33).

- Ironically, when these medicines go down, so do a lot of vitamins and minerals. Among the casualties are: Vitamin K, calcium, magnesium, iron, zinc, vitamin C, vitamin B_2, folic acid, and niacin.
- These medications may make your child more sensitive to sunlight. To prevent bad sunburn, make sure your child avoids too much sun and, when exposed, wears a good sunscreen. (This sunlight sensitivity can continue from 2 weeks to several months after discontinuing the medication.)
- Do not give *tetracyclines* to children under the age of 8 without being specifically directed to do so by a physician.
- If your child is on *tetracycline* antibiotics, be sure that his or her diet has plenty of iron-rich foods (meat, farina, dried peaches, nuts, asparagus, oatmeal), along with high-calcium products such as milk, cheese, soybeans, sardines, peanuts, salmon, sunflower seeds, and green vegetables.
- While your child is on medication, a worthwhile supplement program would be vitamin C (500–1,000 mg.), vitamin B complex (25–50 mg.), and acidophilus (3 caps or 1 tbsp. liquid) daily.

SULFONAMIDES
(GANTANOL, BACTRIM, SEPTRA, GANTRISIN)

- These medicines work best when taken on an empty stomach with a full glass of water.
- Children on this type of medication should drink plenty of water during the day, which helps prevent unwanted side effects.
- RENOQUID (*sulfacytine*) is one sulfonamide that should *not* be given to children under 14 years of age.
- Children taking sulfonamides should avoid too much sun; they could get a bad sunburn quite easily. (In fact, they might remain sensitive to sunlight for several months after discontinuing the medication.)
- These medications are known depleters of vitamin K.

- Make sure your child's meals include lots of yogurt, egg yolks, leafy greens, and alfalfa. (Use safflower oil for cooking.)

PHENOBARBITAL

- If your child is taking pediatric drops, don't use them if the solution becomes cloudy.
- Pediatric drops may be given mixed with milk or juices, but make sure you don't mix them with too much liquid or the child may not get all the medicine.
- This medication can deprive your child of such important nutrients as folic acid, vitamins B_{12}, D, and K.
- While your child is on this medication, plan menus that include tuna, milk, salmon, cantaloupe, eggs, deep-green leafy vegetables, and alfalfa.
- A nutritious and delicious blender drink for kids on *phenobarbital* is 1 cup of milk, ¼ fresh cantaloupe, 1 tsp. honey, 1 tbsp. milk and egg protein powder, and 3 ice cubes.
- A supplement regimen that I'd recommend for the child while on medication is a good vitamin B-complex (which includes niacinamide and magnesium) daily.

73. Avoiding the sugars

A spoonful of sugar might make the medicine go down, but the not-so-sweet truth is that far too many Rx and OTC liquid medicines for kids are loaded with sugar. (A lot more than a spoonful!) As a parent, you should be aware that there are sugar-free medicines available for your children and, in most cases, these medicines can be substituted on request by your doctor or pharmacist for a particular medicine's sugary twin.

SUGAR-FREE MEDICINES

ANTACIDS AND DIGESTANTS

ALUDROX
ALUSCOP
CAMALOX

MILK OF BISMUTH
MYLANTA LIQUID
MYLANTA-II LIQUID

CREAMALIN   MYLICON DROPS
DELCID   PEPTO-BISMOL
DIGESTAMIC   PROBILAGOL LIQUID
DIMACID   RIOPAN SUSPENSION
ESTOMUL-M   ROBALATE ELIXIR
GELUSIL (Plain, Flavor pack)   TITRALAC
KOLANTYL   WINGEL
MAALOX SUSPENSION

ANTIASTHMATICS AND BRONCHODILATORS

ALUPENT SYRUP   NEOTHYLLINE ELIXIR
CO-XAN   NEOTHYLLINE-GG ELIXIR
ELIXOPHYLLIN   SYNOPHYLATE
EPHED-ORGANIDIN ELIXIR   TEDRAL ELIXIR
ISUPREL COMPOUND   TEDRAL PEDIATRIC
  ELIXIR   SUSPENSION
LIXAMINOL   THEO-ORGANIDIN
MUDRANE GG   THEOPHYLLINE ELIXIR

ANTIBIOTICS AND ANTI-INFECTIVES

ANTIMINTH SUSPENSION   NEGGRAM SUSPENSION
COMPOCILLIN-V ORAL   ROBITET SUSPENSION
  SUSPENSION   TERRAMYCIN DROPS
FURADANTIN ORAL   TERRAMYCIN SYRUP
  SUSPENSION   TETRACYN SYRUP
FUROXONE LIQUID   THIOSULFIL SUSPENSION
MANDELAMINE   VIBRAMYCIN SYRUP
  SUSPENSION

ANTICONVULSANTS

MYSOLINE SUSPENSION

ANTIDEPRESSANTS AND STIMULANTS

AVENTYL LIQUID   SINEQUAN ORAL
CENALENE   CONCENTRATE
CORAMINE ORAL
  SOLUTION

ANTIDIARRHEALS

BUTIBEL
COLY-MYCIN PEDIATRIC
 SUSPENSION
CORRECTIVE MIXTURE
CORRECTIVE MIXTURE
 w/PAREGORIC
FUROXONE SUSPENSION
INFANTOL
INFANTOL PINK
KAOLIN-PECTIN
 MIXTURE
KAOLIN-PECTIN
 w/NEOMYCIN
KAOPECTATE
KAOPECTATE
 CONCENTRATE
LOMOTIL
OPIUM TINCTURE
PAREGORIC
PAREPECTOLIN
PECTO-KALIN SUSPENSION

ANTISPASMODICS

BELLADONNA
 ALKALOIDS w/PB ELIXIR
BELLADONNA TINCTURE

COUGH AND COLD PREPARATIONS

CEROSE
CEROSE-DM
CETRO-CIROSE
CIDICOL
CLISTIN EXPECTORANT
COLREX COMPOUND
 ELIXIR
COLREX EXPECTORANT
COLREX SYRUP
CONAR
CORYBAN-D SYRUP
COVANAMINE LIQUID
COVANGESIC LIQUID
CO-XAN
DIMETAPP ELIXIR
HYCOMINE PEDIATRIC
 SYRUP
HYCOMINE SYRUP
ISOCLOR LIQUID
LANATUSS
ORGANIDIN SOLUTION
ORNACOL LIQUID
PRUNICODEINE
ROMILAR III, SYRUP
RYNA-C SYRUP
SORBUTUSS
SPANTUSS
TERPIN HYDRATE &
 CODEINE (Parke-Davis)
TUSSAR SF
TUSSIONEX SUSPENSION
TUSSI-ORGANIDIN
TUSSI-ORGANIDIN DM
TUSS-ORNADE

LAXATIVES AND STOOL SOFTENERS

AGORAL (Plain and Flavored)
CASCARA SAGRADA
  FLUIDEXTRACT
CASTOR OIL
CASTOR OIL (Flavored)
COLACE LIQUID
COLOGEL
HALEY'S M-O
KONDREMUL (Plain)
  w/PHENOLPHTHALEIN
  and w/CASCARA
MAGNESIA & ALUMINA
  ORAL SUSPENSION

MILK OF BISMUTH
MILK OF MAGNESIA
MILK OF MAGNESIA-
  CASCARA SUSPENSION
MILK OF MAGNESIA-
  MINERAL OIL EMULSION
MINERAL OIL
NEOLOID
PERI-COLACE
PHOSPHO-SODA
RECTALAD

MISCELLANEOUS

CĒPACOL
CHLORASEPTIC
DECADRON ELIXIR
GLYCERIN SOLUTION
  (Flavored) 50 percent
KAOCHLOR
  CONCENTRATE
KAOCHLOR S-F
KAON ELIXIR
KAY CIEL ELIXIR

KOLYUM
PARADIONE SOLUTION
POTASSIUM CHLORIDE
  LIQUID
POTASSIUM CHLORIDE
  POWDER
POTASSIUM GLUCONATE
  ELIXIR
POTASSIUM IODIDE LIQUID
TYLENOL DROPS

SEDATIVES, TRANQUILIZERS

AMYTAL ELIXIR
BUTISOL SODIUM ELIXIR
HALDOL CONCENTRATE
MELLARIL CONCENTRATE
  30 mg/ml
PERMITIL ORAL
  CONCENTRATE
PHENOBARBITAL LIQUID
  100 mg/5 ml

SEDADROPS
SERENTIL CONCENTRATE
THORAZINE
  CONCENTRATE
TRICLOS LIQUID
VESPRIN SUSPENSION
VISTARIL SUSPENSION

VITAMINS, MINERALS, LIPOTROPICS

ADEFLOR DROPS
AQUASOL A DROPS
AQUASOL E DROPS
BETALIN COMPLEX
  ELIXIR
C-B TIME
CECON SOLUTION
CE-VI-SOL DROPS
COD LIVER OIL
DRISDOL IN PROPYLENE
  GLYCOL
FERROLIP SYRUP
IBERET-LIQUID
  ORAL SOLUTION
KAOCHLOR S-F TEN
  PERCENT LIQUID
KARIDIUM
KAY CIEL
LIPOMUL-ORAL
LIPOTRIAD

LURIDE DROPS
NIFEREX ELIXIR
PEDIAFLOR
PFIKLOR
PHOS-FLUR ORAL RINSE
POLY-VI-FLOR DROPS
POLY-VI-SOL DROPS
POLY-VI-SOL w/IRON
  DROPS
POTASSIUM CHLORIDE
POTASSIUM GLUCONATE
POTASSIUM TRIPLEX
SUPER D OIL
THERAGRAN LIQUID
TOLERON SUSPENSION
TRI-VI-FLOR DROPS
TRI-VI-SOL w/IRON
  DROPS
VI-DAYLIN/F ADC DROPS

74. Vitamin and medicine facts parents should know

- Children being treated for acne or other dermatological conditions with medications containing large doses of vitamin A can develop chronic hypervitaminosis A (dry skin, hair loss, sore lips, nausea, loss of appetite).
- Be aware of medicines that deplete vitamin B_{12}, because symptoms of a B_{12} deficiency may take as long as *five* years to appear *after* the child's body has been depleted. (Deficiency symptoms usually begin with weakness in arms and legs, diminished reflex response, difficulty in walking and speaking.)
- Antacids (such as TUMS, ROLAIDS, MAALOX, etc.)— when used too often—can deplete a child's system of phosphate and lead to muscle weakness.

- Large amounts of vitamin C can reverse the anticoagulant activity of blood-thinning medications.
- The anticoagulant activity of blood-thinning medications can also be reversed by an excessive intake of leafy vegetables—especially spinach, cauliflower, and brussels sprouts. (The high vitamin C and K content of these foods is responsible for the decrease in the drug's activity.)
- Children with heart disorders should have their vitamin D dosages prescribed by a physician.
- Vitamin E should be given cautiously to any child with an overactive thyroid, diabetes, high blood pressure, or rheumatic heart. (A child with any of these conditions could be started on a very low dosage, which can gradually be increased.)
- A child with rheumatic fever (or rheumatic heart) has an imbalance between the two sides of the heart, and large vitamin E doses can increase the imbalance and worsen the condition. (Consult the child's doctor before using supplements.)
- A youngster with a history of convulsive disorders should not be given large doses of folic acid for any extended period of time.
- Folic acid and PABA can inhibit the effectiveness of sulfonamides, such as GANTRISIN.
- Carrots and liver will not give an effective amount of vitamin A to a child with a zinc deficiency.
- Niacin and supplements that contain it should be given cautiously to children with diabetes, glaucoma, ulcer, or liver problems.
- Iron should not be taken by any child with such blood disorders as sickle-cell anemia, hemochromatosis, or thalassemia.
- Ferrous-sulfate iron supplements can decrease a child's vitamin E.
- Excessive doses of iron-fortified vitamins or OTC medicinal iron formulas can cause iron poisoning in children.
- If your child is taking medication for an underactive thyroid gland, remember that kelp can affect that

gland. (If you've added kelp to the child's diet, he or she might need *less* prescription medicine.)

- Inform the doctor if your child is taking supplementary C, because vitamin C can alter the results of many lab tests.
- Mineral oil, taken internally, can deplete your child of vitamins A, D, E, and K.

75. Any questions about Chapter X?

My two-month-old son is getting nothing but breast milk. Are there any natural foods that will enrich my milk?

Lots. Aside from making sure you're eating nutrient-high balanced meals, you can try adding some herbs to your diet. Powdered marshmallow root and blessed thistle, mixed in juice or milk and drunk several times a day, can enrich mother's milk. (They can also help clear up baby's skin rash.)

Adding brewer's yeast to your diet can aid in increasing the quality as well as the quantity of the milk.

Are there any medicines or vitamins to prevent tooth decay?

The best preventive for tooth decay is limiting your child's intake of sugars and starches (together they create a sticky substance more likely to cling to teeth than sugar alone). But having your child eat a slice of aged cheddar cheese immediately after sugar can help check the beginning of decay.

There is an anticavity vaccine that researchers hope to have perfected by the end of the 1980s, but even this will not give kids license to eat unlimited amounts of sugar.

Diets with plenty of vitamins A, C, and D, calcium, magnesium, and phosphorus, are still important, as is fluoridated drinking water or, in nonfluoridated areas, a fluoride supplement, which should only be given with a doctor's prescription.

What kind of effects would my taking an antibiotic—other than tetracycline—have on my baby while breast-feeding?

It would still depend on the antibiotic, but theoretically it could cause hypersensitivity reactions. Also, it's likely that it would alter the bacterial flora of your child's intestinal tract, which is important to early development of the immune system.

CHAPTER XI

Dieters' Drugs

76. Do they work?

Prescription appetite suppressants such as PRELUDIN, DIDREX, TENUATE, IONAMIN, and others have been shown to be effective in the treatment of obesity *only* on a short-term basis (2 weeks). The same holds true for amphetamines and amphetamine-related drugs, whose value the FDA has deemed "clinically trivial" for dieters in view of their potential for misuse.

> A dieter who uses amphetamines to lose weight usually winds up an overweight person hooked on amphetamines instead of just an overweight person.

Though these drugs suppress the appetite temporarily, tolerance is easily acquired; and after several weeks, doses must be increased to provide the same amount of appetite suppression.

The difference in effectiveness between people who start diets with appetite suppressants and those who start diets with-

out them is so small and short-term, while the risks of drug
dependency and side effects (see section 45) are so great, the
disadvantages in most cases far outweigh the advantages. More
often than not, a dieter who uses amphetamines winds up as an
overweight person hooked on amphetamines instead of merely
an overweight person.

**77. Over-the-counter diet aids: What they are, what they do,
what they don't do**

REDUCING CANDIES

These are supposed to suppress your appetite by being taken
before meals and raising your blood sugar so you won't be as
hungry. Most of these candies (e.g., AYDS) contain about 25
calories apiece (the usual directions specify 2 before each meal),
which means 50 calories, an amount that will produce a negligible effect on your blood sugar level. These candies also include
some vitamins and minerals, and are usually packaged with
exercise and diet regimens, which are probably responsible for
most (if not all) of any weight loss achieved.

BULK-PRODUCING PRODUCTS

Bulk producers, such as the vegetable product *methylcellulose*, are usually taken ten to twenty minutes before meals
and are supposed to swell up in the stomach when they absorb
water and thereby eliminate hunger.

There is no real evidence that these products, which were
originally used to treat constipation, actually reduce hunger
pangs.

BULK PRODUCERS WITH BENZOCAINE

Such products as REDUCETS, SLIM-MINT, and DEXULE
contain *methylcellulose* with *benzocaine*, a topical anesthetic. In
theory, the *benzocaine* is supposed to anesthetize the lining of
the mouth or stomach and in so doing reduce hunger. My
opinion? Save your money and keep away from high-calorie
desserts, junk foods, and other pound putter-oners.

PHENYLPROPANOLAMINE (PPA)

This drug, which has some pharmacological relationship to amphetamine, is used in many OTC reducing products (DEX-ATRIM, DIET-TRIM, HUNGREX, SLENDER-X, PROLA-MINE) as well as in several cold preparations as a nasal decongestant (CORICIDIN-D, SINE-AID, TRIAMINICIN). But as far as PPA being used as a weight reduction aid, the AMA has stated that it's "probably ineffective in the dose provided (25 mg.)."

Aside from being a poor substitute for a good diet, PPA can cause such side effects as dry mouth, nervousness, insomnia, nausea, headache, and high blood pressure. It can also interact adversely with MAO inhibitors (see section 35) and some oral contraceptives.

PHENYLALANINE

This is an essential amino acid (amino acids are the building blocks of protein), cannot be produced by the body, and must be obtained from foods and supplements. It is a neural-transmitter, transmitting its signals between nerve cells and the brain. It can be used as an aid to dieting, because it's turned into norepinephrine and dopamine, which seem to reduce hunger. (Norepinephrine releases a hormone, CCK, which in laboratory experiments has caused rats to get skinnier and skinnier.)

It's found naturally in such protein-rich foods as cottage cheese, soy products, skim dry milk, almonds, peanuts, pumpkin and sesame seeds, and lima and soy beans.

Available in 250–500 mg. tablets, it can aid in appetite control if taken one hour before meals with juice or water (no protein). Many people have found that it also can alleviate those down-in-the-dumps diet blues.

78.   What are starch blockers?

Starch blockers, which were the discovery of Dr. J. John Marshall, are essentially the natural, organic protein substance *phaseolamin*, which is extracted from legumes, such as kidney beans, and inhibits the action of the digestive enzyme alpha amylase that converts starch into calories.

It has no effect on protein, vitamins, minerals, fats, and simple sugars—just starches. For example, if you eat a potato, the vitamins, minerals, and other nutrients of the potato are digested and absorbed normally, but the starch (essentially "empty" calories) is not digested and absorbed. Since 80 percent to 90 percent of the calories in a potato come from starch, you'd get all the vital nutrients but very few calories.

One 500 mg. tablet blocks the absorption of 100 grams of starch, which is the equivalent of approximately 400 calories, more starch than is ordinarily eaten at an average meal.

500 mg. of a starch blocker will nutritionally inhibit the digestion of slightly more starch than is contained in the following quantities of food:

Banana	4 medium
Beans	2 cups
Biscuits	6 medium
Bread	4 slices
Corn (canned)	3 cups
Corn (sweet)	6 ears
Cornflakes	5 cups
Macaroni	2½ cups
Noodles	2½ cups
Peas (fresh)	3 cups
Peas (canned)	3 cups
Potato	4 medium
Rice	2 cups
Spaghetti	3 cups
Squash (mashed)	3 cups
Tapioca dessert	1¼ cups
Wheat flour	1 cup

79. How should a starch blocker be taken?

One tablet should be taken *immediately* before (5 minutes) any meal containing starches—or immediately (5 minutes) after. (If you're eating a low-starch meal, half a tablet may be enough.) I suggest, though, that you eat a well-balanced diet which includes protein, vitamins, minerals, a small amount of fats, sufficient quantities of starch, and adequate amounts of water, if using *phaseolamin*. It's best if you consult your physician or a nutritionally-oriented doctor (see section 167) before beginning a starch-blocker regimen, so that you can be sure you're on the nutritionally correct diet for you.

80. Are there side effects?

The FDA has said that starch blockers may cause diarrhea, cramps, may change the bacteria present in the bowel, and might cause an increase in the size of the pancreas. They've also said that overuse of the product might produce a syndrome in which a person could become very ill and confused. Many nutritionally-oriented doctors, though, feel that taking two acidophilus capsules along with a starch blocker can eliminate most of these side effects.

81. Are starch blockers drugs?

The manufacturers say that they're not, because they're a food product derived from beans, but the FDA says that they are drugs, because they alter the function of the body. At this time, all OTC sales have been suspended. Nonetheless, most nutritionally-oriented physicians still agree with Dr. J. John Marshall that starch blockers are natural, safe, and effective if taken as directed.

82. What is your appestat?

It's nothing like your sign. Actually it's an area of the hypothalamus (part of the brain) which controls your appetite for food, and everyone's is different. According to recent research, the amount of fat cells you have, which were acquired at birth, crave more fat when the stores in these cells fall below a certain level. (The notion—popular a few years ago—that overfed infants would produce extra fat cells, has now been rejected by most scientists, who feel that heredity is the major determinant.)

Glycerol, which is bound and released according to the fat content of a cell, along with the blood level of insulin, informs the brain of the body's fat reserves. But external influences also affect your body's appestat. For example, the taste and smell of sumptuous food can *raise* your appestat, which operates sort of like a thermostat.

Certain drugs, such as amphetamines, can lower your appestat, but only while you're taking those drugs. Once the pills are discontinued, your appestat goes right back up to where it was. (Nicotine can do the same thing.)

But the good news is that exercise and good physical conditioning can lower your appestat—which means it can help you lose weight faster and more effectively than pills or cigarettes.

83. What should you weigh?

Before rushing out to buy diet pills or set off on a crash diet, why not see what the American Medical Association feels is the right weight for you.

HEIGHT	HEALTHY WEIGHT (without clothes)		
	Small frame	Average frame	Large frame
MEN			
5'4"	122	133	145
5'6"	130	142	155
5'8"	139	151	166
5'10"	147	159	174
6'	154	167	183
6'2"	162	175	192
6'3"	165	178	195
WOMEN			
5'	100	109	118
5'2"	107	115	125
5'4"	113	122	132
5'6"	120	129	139
5'8"	126	136	146
5'10"	133	144	156
6'	141	152	166

84. Any questions about Chapter XI?

There are sugar substitutes and starch blockers, but what about fat substitutes? Are there any?

They're not on the market yet, but it shouldn't be long. Researchers at the University of Cincinnati have discovered a synthetic fat substance—containing artificial fat—that your body *won't* absorb.

The synthetic fat, sucrose polyester, was used in a recent test as a substitute for milk fats to create low-calorie milkshakes. It was also used to make salad dressings and a margarine-like spread. Test participants lost an average of four-tenths of a pound a day, and nine out of ten of the participants couldn't tell the difference between the synthetic fat and the real thing. And even better, the synthetic fat can also lower cholesterol levels!

What's the best diet to go on?

The one that's right for YOU! Establish how many calories you need to stay the weight you are, then determine how many you should cut out daily to lose. It takes 3,500 calories to gain or lose a pound. If you're currently eating 2,700 calories daily, all you have to do is cut out 500 calories a day and you should be able to lose 1 pound a week with no trouble. Keep in mind, too, that exercise lowers your craving for food, and helps speed off those extra pounds.

My girlfriend told me that eating algae can help you lose weight. Is this true?

By algae I think she meant the blue-green algae known as spirulina plankton, or, as it's commonly referred to, spirulina. And yes, she's right!

Spirulina—which is 65 percent protein, rich in chelated minerals such as iron, calcium, zinc, potassium, and magnesium, as well as vitamin A and the B-complex vitamins—contains phenylalanine, which acts on the brain's appetite center to decrease hunger. In fact, spirulina does this easily, because its protein is far easier for the body to digest than most proteins, and it also keeps your blood sugar at the proper level.

The FDA has tested spirulina and determined it safe for human use. It comes in 500-mg. tablets or in powder form. Three 500-mg. tablets taken ½ hour before meals can bring startlingly effective results. (You can decrease the dosage to one or two tablets as you begin to shed pounds.) Some people require six to eight tablets before meals, but I'd advise consulting a nutritionally-oriented doctor if you find this is the case.

CHAPTER XII

Habit-Forming Drugs

85. How you get hooked

The one thing to keep in mind when taking any medicine, be it Rx or OTC, is if it gives you a lift, mellows you out, puts you to sleep, or alters your state of consciousness, *it can be habit-forming!*

Drug habits are formed in several ways:

PHYSICAL DEPENDENCE

This means that the drug's pharmacological properties affect your body in such a way that you develop a physical compulsion to take the drug on a continuous or periodic basis in order to experience its effects and/or avoid the discomfort of its absence—withdrawal symptoms.

PSYCHOLOGICAL DEPENDENCE

Though the drug is not truly addictive in the physical sense, because of its stimulant, sedative, analgesic, or mind-altering properties, you develop a very real compulsion to take it on a continuous or periodic basis—in other words, it becomes a habit.

DRUG TOLERANCE

Any drug that you develop a tolerance for with repeated usage (meaning that you must take more and more of it to achieve the original desired effect) can be habit-forming and potentially dangerous.

86. Drugs that can be habit-forming

(NOTE: The following is a significant but not a complete list, so be sure to ask your pharmacist about the potential for addiction of every medicine you take.)

ALL NARCOTICS

• drugs containing *opium, morphine, codeine, heroin*

SYNTHETIC NARCOTICS

• *hydromorphone hydrochloride* (DILAUDID, DILAUDID COUGH SYRUP)
• *levorphanol tartrate* (LEVO-DROMORAN)
• *meperidine hydrochloride* (DEMEROL)
• *oxycodone hydrochloride* (PERCOCET-5, PERCODAN, PER-CODAN-DEMI, TYLOX)
• *pentazocine hydrochloride* (TALWIN)
• *propoxyphene hydrochloride* (DARVON, PROPOX 65 w/ APAP, SK-65, WYGESIC)
• *propoxyphene napsylate* (DARVOCET-N)

STIMULANTS/APPETITE SUPPRESSANTS
(amphetamine and amphetamine-related drugs)

• *benzphetamine hydrochloride* (DIDREX)
• *chlorphentermine* (PRE-SATE)
• *diethylpropion* (TENUATE, TEPANIL)
• *mazindol* (SANOREX)
• *phendimetrazine* (BONTRIL, PDM, PLEGINE)
• *phenmetrazine* (PRELUDIN)
• *phentermine hydrochloride* (ADIPEX-P, FASTIN, T-DIET, TERAMINE)
• *phentermine resin* (IONAMIN)

SEDATIVES/TRANQUILIZERS/HYPNOTICS

- all barbiturates (ALURATE ELIXIR, AMYTAL, BUFF-A COMP TABS, BUTICAPS, BUTISOL, MEBARAL, NEMBUTAL, PENTOTHOL, PHENOBARBITAL, PLEXONAL, SECONAL, TUINAL)
- *butalbital* (AMAPHEN, FIORINAL, G-2 CAPSULES, G-3 CAPSULES, MEDIGESIC PLUS, PACAPS, PHRENILLIN, REPAN, ROGESIC, SEDAPAP-10, T-GESIC)
- benzodiazepines (ATIVAN, DALMANE, CENTRAX, LIBRIUM, SERAX, VALIUM, VERSTRAN)
- *meprobamate* (DEPROL, EQUAGESIC, EQUANIL, MEPROCON, MEPROSPAN, MICRAININ, MILPATH, MILTOWN, PMB-200, PATHIBAMATE, SK-BAMATE)
- others (NOCTEC, QUAALUDE, PLACIDYL, DORIDEN)

ANTISPASMODICS/ANTICHOLINERGICS

- *atropine sulfate* (ANTROCOL)
- *phenobarbital & other ingredients* (DONNATAL, KINESED)
- *chlordiazepoxid hydrochloride* (LIBRAX)

ANTIMIGRAINE PREPARATIONS

(also used for menstrual & stomach problems)

- *erogotamine tartrate* (BELLERGAL, BELLERGAL S, BELLERMINE O.D., CAFERGOT, ERGOMAR, ERGOSTAT, GYNERGEN, MIGRAL, WIGRAINE)

LAXATIVES

- *phenolphthalein* (AGORAL, EVAC-Q-KWICK, SAROLAX, TRILAX), or any stimulant laxative, can lead to rebound constipation and may cause laxative dependency (see section 48).

Beware, too, of OTC nasal decongestants which, if used often, create a "rebound" cycle. This happens because when the drug wears off, the nasal membranes swell even more and are eventually unable to shrink without higher and higher doses. The same can hold true for eye drops that shrink blood vessels in the eyes.

For all OTC medications, READ LABELS! Far too many still contain large amounts of caffeine, which is a drug, and a habit-forming one!

87. Foods and supplements that can break bad habits

If you realize that you're hooked (see section 85) on a medication and want to get unhooked, it's not advisable to go "cold turkey." Withdrawal symptoms can be uncomfortable and even dangerous. It's best to discuss your problem with a doctor, but if that isn't possible, my advice is to decrease your intake of the drug slowly and fortify yourself with a nutritionally power-packed diet and a nerve-soothing supplement program.

Your habit breaking diet should include:

- Foods high in B-complex vitamins (nutritional yeast, liver, leafy green vegetables, cheese, fish, eggs)
- Lots of vitamin C-rich foods (citrus fruits, strawberries, tomatoes, cauliflower, green and leafy vegetables)
- Calcium aplenty (milk, milk products, cheese, soybeans, peanuts, walnuts, dried beans, green vegetables)
- Foods containing folic acid (carrots, cantaloupe, whole wheat and dark rye flour)
- The best natural sources of tryptophan (milk, natural cheeses, turkey, and bananas)

Avoid:

- Refined and processed sugars and foods that contain them.
- Foods with artificial coloring.
- Foods containing sodium nitrate or sodium nitrite.
- Foods containing the additives MSG (monosodium glutamate), BHT, and BHA.

SUGGESTED SUPPLEMENTS

High-potency multiple vitamin A.M. & P.M.
with chelated minerals
(time-release)

Vitamin C	500–1,000 mg. 2 to 3 times daily
Vitamin B-complex	100 mg. 3 times daily
Vitamin E	200–400 IU 2 to 3 times daily
Acidophilus	3 caps or 2 tbsp. liquid 3 times daily
Lecithin granules	1 tbsp. or 3 1200 mg. caps 3 times daily
Chelated calcium & magnesium	1 tablet 2 to 3 times daily
Tryptophan	250–667 mg. 1 to 3 times daily; take with water or juice (no protein)

88. Any questions about Chapter XII?

Is it possible to become physically addicted to a food?

Yes, indeed. Any food or beverage that contains caffeine can become physically addicting. In fact, studies have shown that people who consume large amounts of coffee daily and then suddenly switch to decaffeinated brands suffer withdrawal symptoms. The same can happen to "chocoholics" who break their sweet habit abruptly.

Can you become addicted to a drug if you take it exactly as your doctor prescribed?

Definitely! Substances that are physically or psychologically addicting remain so even when taken precisely as directed. In fact, if you're taking any of the drugs listed in section 86, it's important to discuss the possibility of withdrawal symptoms with your doctor before discontinuing the medication.

CHAPTER XIII

Illicit and Abused Drugs

89. What they are

Illicit and abused drugs (sometimes referred to as "recreational drugs") are legal and illegal drugs that are obtained and used for other than medicinal purposes—or at least not for the medicinal purposes for which they were originally intended.

MOST COMMONLY ABUSED DRUGS

Alcohol (see sections 156–160)

Amphetamines (e.g., BENZEDRINE, DEXEDRINE, PRELUDIN, RITALIN)

Amyl nitrite

Barbiturates (e.g., AMYTAL, LUMINAL, NEMBUTAL, PHENO-BARBITAL, SECONAL, TUINAL)

Belladonna

Benzodiazepines (e.g., ATIVAN, DALMANE, LIBRIUM, VALIUM)

Caffeine

Cocaine

Codeine

DARVON

DEMEROL

DILAUDID

DORIDEN

ELAVIL

Hashish

Hash oil

Heroin
Inhalants (glue-sniffing)
LSD
Marijuana
MDA
Meprobamate (EQUANIL,
   MILTOWN)
Mescaline
Methadone
Methaqualone
Morphine
Nicotine (see sections
   161–166)
Nitrous oxide
NOCTEC
NOLUDAR
Opium

PARAL
Paregoric
PCP
PERCODAN
Peyote
Phenothiazines (e.g.,
   COMPAZINE,
   MELLARIL,
   STELAZINE,
   THORAZINE)
PLACIDYL
Psilocybin
STP
THC
TRIAVIL
VALMID

90. Some hard, fast facts about amphetamines

SOME STREET NAMES

Bennies, black beauties, blackbirds, crystal, dexies, double-cross, greenies, hearts, lidpoppers, meth, pep pills, skyrockets, sparkle plenties, uppers, whites

WHAT YOU SHOULD KNOW

Amphetamines stimulate the central nervous system and produce adrenalin-like effects which cause your heart, blood, and pulse pressure to rise, and get all your bodily systems going at high speed. They're usually taken orally and are quickly assimilated into the bloodstream, but they may also be sniffed, injected intravenously, smoked, or "skin-popped" (subcutaneous injection).

Effects last from 4 to 14 hours (depending on dosage), and the drug can be detected in blood and urine lab tests up to 72 hours after ingestion. Effects are characterized by

- dilated pupils
- rapid breathing, heartbeat, and speech

- increased wakefulness and alertness
- feelings of increased initiative and ability
- euphoria
- depression of appetite

DANGERS

When the drug begins to wear off, nervousness, paranoia, and fatigue set in, along with headache and palpitations. (The syndrome is known as "crashing.") Because of this, most users feel that the only remedy is to take more amphetamine. Since tolerance can develop quickly, more and more of the drug is needed to produce the original effect.

A single large dose or repeated small doses over an extended period of time can cause a toxic reaction (amphetamine psychosis) which can last from several days to several weeks.

Heavy users of speed can develop tremors or malnutrition, and can acquire an increased susceptibility to infection and disease.

Memory loss and delusions may exist up to a year after the drug is discontinued.

FOODS AND VITAMINS THAT CAN HELP

Niacinamide and vitamin C—1,000 mg. of each—taken after each meal can help restore energy levels and alleviate the discomforts of a hard comedown ("crash").

A nutritious calcium-rich diet (see section 55), along with plenty of liquids and a high-potency multiple vitamin with chelated minerals (taken 1 to 3 times daily), can help speed users get back on a healthy drug-free track.

91. The lowdown on "downers"—barbiturates

SOME STREET NAMES

Barbs, blue devils, downers, goofballs, goofers, green dragons, nemmies, phennies, pink ladies, rainbows, red devils, reds, sleepers, tooies, yellow jackets, yellows

WHAT YOU SHOULD KNOW

The legitimate uses of barbiturates are explained in section 50. But used illicitly as "downers," these drugs, which are CNS depressants, are used as escapes into a tension-free, soft-around-the-edges, carefree world. Sometimes these drugs are used in combination with amphetamines ("speedballing"), either taken together or one after the other. The results can create separate addictions, and create a vicious cycle that often winds up at a literal *dead* end.

DANGERS

The dangers of barbiturate abuse are many and serious, especially with long-term use. Chronic symptoms that commonly develop are

- shortened memory
- constant drowsiness
- loss of coordination and awareness
- emotional instability
- slurred speech
- paranoia

A big danger with barbiturate abuse is drug tolerance, because while you need more and more of the drug to achieve the desired effect, *the lethal dosage remains the same!* (A lethal dose is estimated at ten times the prescribed dosage.)

An even bigger danger is combining barbiturates with alcohol. *This can be deadly!* Even a small amount of barbiturates with alcohol can cause an overdose.

Withdrawal symptoms are severe, even more than from heroin. They usually begin with anxiety and become increasingly violent, and—depending upon how hooked the user is—can result in seizures and even death. Withdrawal should definitely be done under medical supervision.

FOODS AND VITAMINS THAT CAN HELP

Whether you're taking downers or breaking the habit, increasing your B vitamins can help. Be sure your diet includes foods high in calcium, niacin, and choline as well. (See section 55.) For supplements, I'd advise vitamin B-complex, 100 mg. 3 times daily; tryptophan 250–667 mg. 2 to 3 times daily; a high-potency multiple vitamin with chelated minerals (time release) A.M. and P.M.; and niacinamide 100–500 mg. 1 to 3 times daily along with vitamin C, 1,000 mg.

92. Cocaine is expensive in more ways than you think

SOME STREET NAMES

Blow, coke, dream dust, flakes, nose candy, snow, toot, white

WHAT YOU SHOULD KNOW

Cocaine is a vasoconstrictor, a stimulant of the central nervous system, and potentiates the effects of nerve stimulation. When applied externally, it blocks impulse conduction in nerve fibers and produces a numbing effect.

Though it comes in the forms of rock, flake, and powder, it's the latter that is most available—though it's rarely more than 60 percent pure cocaine. The rest is the "cut," which is used by dealers to dilute or enhance the drug for more profit.

Some cuts are pharmacologically inert, such as lactose, dextrose, inositol (a B vitamin), and mannitol. These in themselves are relatively harmless, but other nondrug "cuts" such as cornstarch, talcum powder, and flour can be dangerous because they are basically insoluble in blood and can clot up in the body.

Other cuts, which are pharmacologically active and usually other local anesthetics, are *procaine*, *lidocaine*, and *benzocaine*. *Benzocaine*, though, is relatively insoluble and can cause blood clots and serious complications if injected. Stimulants such as *methamphetamine*, BENZEDRINE, and DEXEDRINE—among others—are also used as "cuts" to enhance the potency of the cocaine.

Nasal inhalation of cocaine is the most popular form of taking the drug. Because it is absorbed rapidly through the mucous membranes, it is also often applied locally under the eyelids and tongue, and on the genital region. Cocaine can also be injected intravenously or smoked in a process called "free basing."

Its effects are euphoria, feelings of intense psychic energy and self-confidence, and, as with amphetamines, a loss of appetite. But these effects are short-lived (about ½ hour), and more coke is necessary to recapture the high. The drug is not physically addictive, but psychological dependence is high.

DANGERS

This expensive drug draws a lot from your body as well as your bankbook. With repeated large doses, any or all of the following can occur:

- Nosebleeding
- Increased heartbeat
- The feeling that ants or bugs are crawling on or under your skin
- Cold sweats
- Nausea, vomiting, and an increase in body temperature
- Convulsions
- Anaphylactic shock

The biggest danger involved in using cocaine is that its toxicity is unpredictable. Even small doses with the wrong cut can cause serious problems in individuals with varying sensitivities. Cocaine poisoning, which can result in immediate death, is usually caused by too rapid absorption of the drug—usually through intravenous injection.

FOODS AND VITAMINS THAT CAN HELP

Even if your pocketbook can afford this drug, your body can't. Because it is an appetite depressant, you're probably skipping meals and losing needed nutrients, especially stress vitamins B and C. And even if you're an infrequent user, your nasal tissues need all the help they can get.

I'd strongly recommend a good multiple-vitamin and mineral tablet and a high-potency multiple mineral be taken twice daily, along with vitamin C, 1,000 mg., vitamin E, 200–400 IU, and vitamin B-complex, 100 mg. 1 to 3 times daily.

93. Marijuana and hashish

SOME STREET NAMES

Boo, bush, Columbian, dope, ganja, gold, goof butt, grass, Hawaiian, hay, hemp, herb, J, joint, kif, Maryjane, pod, pot, reefer, rope, shit, smoke, stick, tea, weed

WHAT YOU SHOULD KNOW

Marijuana and hashish come from the hemp plant *cannabis sativa*. The marijuana consists of the chopped leaves and stems of the plant, while the hashish is formed from the resin scraped from the flowering tops. The psychoactive ingredient in both these drugs is delta-9-tetrahydrocannabinol (THC). Neither drug is an hallucinogen or a sedative, but they share characteristics of both.

Marijuana and hashish can be either smoked or eaten. If smoked, the effects—depending on the quality of drugs and the metabolism of the individual—last for 1 to 3 hours. If eaten, they can last from 4 to 10 hours, though it takes longer (about an hour) for the user to feel them.

Unlike other illicit drugs, marijuana and hashish seem to have the curious property of "reverse tolerance," which means that seasoned users need less of the drug to get high than first-timers. This is probably caused by THC accumulating in the body, requiring only a small additional amount for a regular user to achieve an effect.

Though the chemical and psychological effects of these drugs vary with the individual, they essentially act as relaxants, tranquilizers, appetite stimulants, intoxicants, enhancers of the senses, and mild hallucinogens.

DANGERS

Serious adverse reactions to marijuana are rare, and are much more common when hashish, which is more powerful, is used. Such reactions are:

- Depression (usually an intensification of a preexisting mood)

- Panic (usually in users without prior drug experience)
- Toxic psychosis (can occur if *cannabis* is eaten and the user hasn't been able to judge amount ingested)
- Psychotic reactions (risk high only in users with preexisting mental disorders)
- Smoking marijuana, though, does raise blood pressure and can increase the risk of lung cancer.
- Smoking marijuana during pregnancy can cause low birth weight in newborns.

FOODS AND SUPPLEMENTS THAT CAN HELP

If you're a pot smoker, chances are that you've gotten the "munchies" more than a few times and have had more than your share of refined sugars and carbohydrates, meaning you've deprived yourself of necessary B vitamins. And the smoking of one joint can lower the vitamin C level in your blood.

All smoking is bad for you (see sections 161–166), and marijuana smoking has the added disadvantage of getting you in trouble with the law. But if you do smoke, be sure to increase your intake of citrus fruits and green leafy vegetables. I'd also recommend taking a vitamin C supplement, 1,000 mg. (time-release) morning and night. Also, it would be wise to take vitamin E, 100–400 IU 1 to 3 times daily to protect your lungs.

94. The "heavy" narcotics: morphine, heroin, methadone and meperidine (DEMEROL)

SOME STREET NAMES

Morphine (cube, hard stuff, morf, white stuff); heroin (brown sugar, dope, goods, H, hard stuff, Harry, horse, junk, scag, schmeck, smack, sugar, white stuff); methadone (medicine, dollies, biscuits); DEMEROL (demis, junk, white stuff)

WHAT YOU SHOULD KNOW

Heroin, the main narcotic of abuse in America, is produced by chemical treatment of morphine with acetic acid. It is three times as potent as morphine, breaks down into morphine in the body and, therefore, its pharmacological action is the same.

Methadone is a synthetic narcotic and approximately the same strength as morphine.

Meperidine (DEMEROL) is also a synthetic narcotic, but only about 10 to 20 percent as potent as morphine.

All these narcotics, which are opiates, can be taken orally; sniffed through the nasal passages; "skin-popped" (subcutaneous injection); or injected intravenously (mainlining) or intra-muscularly.

The main desired effect of these drugs, for addicts, is an analgesic euphoria. Opiates cause a mental clouding, a drowsi-ness, an inability to concentrate, and impaired vision, though they do not cause the slurred speech and loss of motor coordi-nation that occurs with alcohol and many other abused drugs.

The most sought-after effect is the "rush" or initial impact of these drugs when injected, which is often described as "orgasmic"; the next most sought-after effect is to ward off the cramps, hot flushes, itchy skin, and chills which occur when the drug begins wearing off and the addict craves another "fix."

DANGERS

Tolerance for these drugs is easily acquired, and more and more of the drug is required not only to achieve the original effect, but to stave off the discomforts of withdrawal. And because these drugs are so closely related, tolerance to one drug is usually transferred to tolerance of the others.

Users who inject these drugs are subject to many illnesses that can be caused by dirty or shared needles. Among them:

- Serum hepatitis
- Blood poisoning
- Tetanus
- Gangrene
- Lockjaw
- Cardiovascular and lung abnormalities

Because these drugs suppress the coughing reflex, users are subject to pneumonia and chronic bronchitis.

Substances that are used to "cut" heroin can cause pulmonary edema, shock, respiratory failure, and death. But what probably contributes most to fatalities among users is injecting the drug while the user is drunk or sedated with barbiturates.

FOODS AND SUPPLEMENTS THAT CAN HELP

Narcotic addicts are generally in poor physical condition, suffering from malnutrition and chronic constipation. If you're hooked on any of these substances, the first thing I'd advise is medical help. Your state department of health or division of substance abuse services can direct you. In the interim, the best you can do for yourself is try to nutritionally rehabilitate your body.

Check section 55 for foods that are your best sources of B vitamins, including choline, folic acid, inositol, and niacin; vitamin C, vitamin E, calcium, magnesium, phosphorus, potassium, and zinc. Supplements are essential, but you have to remember that they are *not* substitutes for food. I'd recommend the following regimen:

High-potency multiple mineral	A.M. & P.M.
Vitamin C	1,000 mg. 3 times daily
Vitamin E	200–400 IU 1 to 3 times daily
Vitamin B-complex	100 mg. 3 times daily
Unprocessed bran flakes	2 tbsp. daily
Bran tablets	3 to 9 daily
Acidophilus liquid	1 tbsp. 3 times daily

95. QUAALUDES

SOME STREET NAMES

Ludes, quacks, quads, 714s, soapers

WHAT YOU SHOULD KNOW

QUAALUDES are nonbarbiturate sedative-hypnotics and act on a different central nervous system site than other sleeping pills, such as barbiturates. They're distributed in body fat, brain tissue, and the liver, and, by reducing neural transmissions to the brain, they suppress REM (rapid eye movement) during dreams, causing deep, though not necessarily restful sleep. They're fast-acting, but users (or rather abusers) of this drug fight the drowsiness that occurs within ten to twenty minutes, seeking the body-relaxing effects. These effects also include being relaxed to the point of noncoordination and being unable to speak without slurring words.

Though touted as having aphrodisiacal qualities, heavy doses have the opposite effect. Though still available on prescription in some states, many states have now outlawed the drug.

Addiction, meaning physical and psychological dependence, is possible within two weeks at a daily dosage of 300–600 mg. All it takes for an overdose is eight 300 mg. tablets.

DANGERS

Users have a tendency to underestimate or misjudge the potency of this drug—or simply forget what they've taken. The biggest danger is the combined effect of QUAALUDES and alcohol, which, because of the synergistic action of the two drugs, can easily lead to overdose. Symptoms are:

- Convulsions
- Tremors
- Stomach hemorrhage

Medical attention is a must, and if overdose is suspected, that attention must be immediate. Keep the victim awake at all costs!

FOODS AND SUPPLEMENTS THAT CAN HELP

Withdrawal from "ludes" is similar to withdrawal from heroin and barbiturates. See section 94 for diet and supplement suggestions that can help you get back on your feet.

96. LSD and other hallucinogens

SOME STREET NAMES

LSD (acid, blotter, Lucy in the sky with diamonds, microdots, white lightning, wedgies); mescaline (buttons, cactus, mesc); psilocybin and psilocin (magic mushrooms)

WHAT YOU SHOULD KNOW

LSD is a synthetic drug and *ergotamine tartate* (the main ingredient in CAFERGOT, ERGOMAR, and ERGOSTAT) can be used as the raw material in its manufacture. Gram for gram it is the most powerful drug known.

Mescaline, which is an alkaloid of the peyote cactus, is not as potent as LSD in altering states of consciousness, but it can still cause grand illusions, fantasies—and bad trips.

Psilocybin and psilocin are about 1 percent as potent as LSD and are the active alkaloids of about twenty types of mushrooms native to Mexico and the southern part of the United States.

LSD is usually taken orally (though it can be snorted or injected). One hundred micrograms are all that are necessary for an eight- to ten-hour hallucinogenic trip. Its first effects are like those of *ephedrine*—pupil dilation, increased blood pressure, tremors, nausea, and so on. These occur about an hour after ingestion. After that, perceptions are altered; afterimages are prolonged, objects seem to melt, and sensory impressions are vivid. A state where colors are "heard" and music is "seen" is common, as is the loss of time perception and the increase of self-perception. The effects of other hallucinogens are similar, although usually less potent.

DANGERS

Bad "trips" which are characterized by extreme panic reactions can occur in anyone. The tranquilizer *chlorpromazine* can often counter these effects, but not always. LSD and other hallucinogens can also produce

- serious depression
- prolonged psychotic episodes
- flashback (a recurrence of some aspect of the drug experience—not necessarily pleasant—when the user is no longer under the drug's influence)

Tolerance to hallucinogens can develop rapidly if the drugs are taken regularly, but there is no physical dependence or withdrawal symptoms. It has been shown, though, that LSD can damage white blood-cell chromosomes.

Perhaps the greatest danger is that because LSD is illegal, it is often sold on the street adulterated with other dangerous chemicals, such as PCP (angel dust), a veterinary anesthetic that can cause not only bad trips but deadly ones.

FOODS AND SUPPLEMENTS THAT CAN HELP

Because these drugs produce effects resembling those resulting from stimulation of the sympathetic nervous system, the regimens suggested for amphetamines in section 90 are applicable here.

97. "LOADS"—the dangerous new drug craze

One of the most lethal drug habits to hit the streets is something called "loads," a combination of two easily-obtained prescription drugs—DORIDEN (a sleeping pill) and *codeine* (a pain-killer). Combined, their effect is stronger than heroin and ten times more addicting—and far deadlier. Because of the potent soporific effects of combining a sedative-hypnotic with codeine, going into a coma is not uncommon—nor is *not coming out of it.*

Withdrawal is similar to that of heroin withdrawal, and medical supervision is vital. See section 94.

98. Any questions about Chapter XIII?

Are there any legal "natural" ways to get high?
There are quite a few, but I don't recommend them. For example, the leaves from the coleus plant can be chewed or

steeped in warm water to make a sort of tea which produces psychedelic effects, and the leaves of the passion flower vine can be dried and smoked for a mild marijuana-like high. But passion flower vine contains alkaloids much like MAO inhibitors, meaning that the same cautions are advised for its use (see section 35); and not enough research has been done on the coleus plant or other legal natural substances used as recreational drugs to guarantee their safety. Why not try getting high on physical and nutritional fitness? That's a *real* buzz!

I've heard about a cocaine substitute that's legal. Is there such a product?

There is a product called TOOT, which looks like cocaine, has a name which is slang for cocaine, but is in reality *phenylpropanolamine* (PPA), *benzocaine*, and *caffeine*. All the ingredients are legal and are found in many OTC products, but that doesn't mean they're safe. *Phenylpropanolamine,* which is in many OTC cold preparations and diet pills, is a CNS stimulant and can cause acute anxiety, hallucinations, tachycardia, and other adverse side effects. Also, if this product is heated, the fumes can be toxic. My advice for playing with this product is play it safe and stay away from it!

CHAPTER XIV

Drugs and VD

99. Genital herpes

Genital herpes, which has reached epidemic proportions in the United States, is a painful rash located on the skin or inner membranes of the vagina, penis, or anus. Caused by a virus, genital herpes is transmitted mainly through sexual contact.

On first contracting herpes, victims find the infection may be accompanied by a high fever, even inflammation of the membranes surrounding the brain and spinal cord (meningitis). The symptoms usually disappear in about two weeks, but, ironically, the virus does not. Instead, it remains latent until some other event (infection, fever, emotional stress, fatigue) reactivates it and causes it to travel down the nerve fibers to again produce pain and rash at the original site.

Once you have a primary herpes infection, it may occur repeatedly, recur a few times and then stop, or simply lie dormant in the body nerve tissues and not produce symptoms for a lifetime. But there's always the chance that it can be reactivated by stress, and it's more than likely to be reactivated upon physical contact with another person with active genital herpes.

100. Help for herpes

Although some viral illnesses can be prevented with vaccines, herpes isn't one of them. At least not yet! In fact, some doctors have endangered their patients' lives by attempting to treat herpes with smallpox vaccine. No matter what you've heard on the herpes grapevine, the Immunization Practices Advisory Committee of the Public Health Service has stated emphatically that "there is no evidence that smallpox vaccination has therapeutic value in the treatment of recurrent herpes . . . and smallpox vaccine should never be used therapeutically."

On the other hand, the New York State Health Department has genetically modified a smallpox vaccine virus that they hope will lead to the first successful vaccine against herpes simplex type I (which causes cold sores and other upper body infections), and that may become the model for other vaccines, including one for type II herpes, which causes genital infection.

But there is even more hope on the herpes horizon! A report in the *American Journal of Obstetrics and Gynecology* has stated the spermicides, such as ORTHO-GYNOL, DELFEN, and EMKO, used with a diaphragm have a protective effect against herpes virus for women. Although not yet tested against placebos (inactive substances used to compare test results), large dietary intakes of the amino acid lysine have been recommended as effective therapy for herpes infections for both sexes. As far as I'm concerned, it couldn't hurt.

FOODS HIGH IN LYSINE

DAIRY PRODUCTS

Cottage cheese (uncreamed) 1 cup	3,584 mg.
Egg—1 med.	406 mg.
Milk, skim, dry, instant—1 cup	1,780 mg.

FISH

Flounder, baked—1 lb.	11,880 mg.
Salmon, pink, canned—1 lb.	8,081 mg.
Shrimp, cooked—1 lb.	7,225 mg.
Tuna, canned, drained—1 lb.	11,504 mg.

FRUITS

Fig, raw—1 med.   117 mg.
Avocado   240 mg.
Strawberries—1 cup   48 mg.

MEATS, POULTRY

Liver, fried—1 lb.   6,772 mg.
Beef, rump roast—1 lb.   8,526 mg.
Lamb—1 lb.   9,543 mg.
Ham, roasted—1 lb.   7,807 mg.

NUTS AND SEEDS

Almonds, dried—1 cup   774 mg.
Peanuts, roasted with skin—1 cup   2,592 mg.
Pumpkin & squash kernels—1 cup   3,068 mg.

VEGETABLES

Green beans—1 cup   104 mg.
Bean sprouts (mung)—1 cup   218 mg.
Cauliflower, raw—1 cup   151 mg.
Chick peas (garbanzos), dry raw—½ cup   1,415 mg.
Green peas (cooked)—1 cup   338 mg.
Soybeans, cooked—1 cup   1,518 mg.

BREAD

Pumpernickel—1 slice   119 mg.

FLOUR

Soy—1 cup   2,784 mg.

101. Syphilis

Syphilis is caused by a tiny corkscrew-like organism called a spirochete. It is usually transmitted by sexual contact and requires only the presence of an open wound or slightly irritated mucous membrane, such as the mouth, rectum, or outer male and female genital organs, to enter the body. (Yes, it can be transmitted through the sputum, after kissing, but this *is* rare.)

First stage symptoms: A painless sore on the penis or the entrance to the vagina 3 to 4 weeks after intercourse with an infected person. (The sore might appear instead or also on the nipple, anus, or finger.)

Second stage symptoms: These occur about 1 to 2 months later. There is a mild general illness, sore throat, mild fever, and a pink nonitchy rash. Laryngitis might be noticed.

Third stage symptoms: These appear four or more years later and are quite rare, as the disease is usually diagnosed by then. But at this point, any organ may be affected and dangerously jeopardized.

If early treatment is started with penicillin or any of the other newer antibiotics, recovery is swift and complete. But some of these remedies cause almost as much need for supplements as the disease itself, which is why I recommend the following:

- High-potency multiple vitamin with chelated minerals (time-release)
- Vitamin C, 1,000 mg.
- High-potency chelated multiple minerals (All A.M. and P.M. with food)

Also: 3 acidophilus capsules 3 times daily, and vitamin K, 100 mcg. daily, if on an extended antibiotic program.

102. Gonorrhea—it's nothing to clap about

Like syphilis, gonorrhea is usually transmitted through sexual contact, but the responsible organism—the gonococcus—has the ability to acquire a resistance to some of the most powerful medical weapons, such as sulfa drugs, *penicillin,* and many of the 'mycins.

Symptoms: These occur 3 to 10 days after infection. There is usually pain on passing urine and a discharge of pus. Often, these symptoms go unnoticed by women.

Early and adequate treatment with antibiotics is essential in order to avoid complications. If the strain is resistant to *penicillin,* there are still *tetracyclines, erythromycin,* and other antibiotics that are effective.

While on any of these drugs, I'd suggest you follow the supplement regimen suggested for syphilis in section 101.

103. Gay Bowel Syndrome

"Gay Bowel Syndrome" is not a disease but merely a term that is now being used to cover a variety of gastrointestinal tract infections that are on the increase among homosexual men and present special diagnostic and treatment considerations because the homosexual transmission of these infections is not generally covered in most medical textbooks.

- Syphilis and gonorrhea are common in gay communities, but because the infection is usually rectal or asymptomatic (and because patients rarely reveal their sexual orientation to the physician), the diseases are often treated incorrectly.
- Hepatitis A and B infections, also common in gay areas, often occur without jaundice and only nonspecific gastrointestinal symptoms.
- Amebiasis, which is venereally transmitted in gay communities, is generally an asymptomatic infection that poses a serious health threat, though it can be effectively treated with YODOXIN and IODOQUINOL (*diiodohydroxyquin*).
- Giardiasis, another sexually-transmitted disease, is often misdiagnosed as a functional bowel disease, when in reality the drug of choice to cure it would probably be ATABRINE (*quinacrine*).
- Shigellosis, a disease characterized by fever, diarrhea, and prostration, is usually self-limiting in heterosexual groups, but in the sexually active male homosexual community antibiotic therapy is necessary. Either *ampicillin* or *TMX sulfa* is usually effective.

The reasons for the rise of these diseases in the homosexual community seem to be primarily the practice of oral-rectal sex, gay baths, and the fact that these diseases have a "carrier" state, meaning a period during which the patient is seemingly healthy but can still transmit the disease.

If you think you have or are carrying any of these diseases, it's important to tell your doctor of your homosexual activities, so that you can get the right treatment for your illness. Foods and supplements recommended in section 54 can help alleviate many of the discomforting symptoms while you're getting well.

104. Any questions about Chapter XIV?

I can't believe that modern science hasn't come up with a drug to fight herpes. Haven't they found any that are effective?

Viruses are tricky, but yes, there are some drugs that look promising. In fact, a relatively new drug called *acyclovir* has been shown to be partially effective for treating herpes infections of the skin and mucous membranes. It is available in three forms: an ointment, a pill, and an intravenous solution. Right now, the ointment, has only limited value. It's only effective when applied early during a *first* episode of genital herpes, where it reduces the severity of local symptoms, but it does not prevent recurrence. The good news is that no serious side effects have been reported for the drug; the bad news is that widespread or extended use may cause a buildup of resistance to its effects.

There is also a new spermicide with a cottonseed oil extract being developed by the Ford Foundation that apparently kills genital herpes virus as well as sperm, but the product has not yet been used in human clinical trials.

Someone told me that mononucleosis can be caused by the herpes virus. Is this true?

Yes, it is. But what you have to understand is that there are five types of herpes viruses, and they can all cause different diseases.

Herpes simplex, type 1, for instance, can be responsible for cold sores, an eye infection known as herpes keratitis, and a brain infection (herpes encephalitis). Herpes simplex, type 2, is the virus responsible for genital herpes and the generalized infection of newborns who are exposed to herpes during childbirth. The herpes virus known as varicella-zoster can cause chicken pox and shingles, and the Epstein-Barr virus is the one responsible for infectious mononucleosis. Cytomegalovirus (CMV) can cause pneumonia in susceptible individuals, as well as a condition which resembles mononucleosis in young adults, recipients of blood transfusions, and many homosexual men.

If foods that are high in lysine can help prevent herpes, are there also foods that could have the opposite effect?

There's nothing definite yet, but researchers seem to feel that foods which contain more of the amino acid arginine than lysine should be avoided. Such foods are—among others—chocolate, popcorn, carob, gelatin desserts, brown rice, oatmeal, raisins, and sesame seeds.

My gynecologist prescribed FLAGYL for my vaginal infection, but I've heard that the drug is unsafe. What's the story?

FLAGYL is the drug of choice for vaginal infections caused by trichomonads (a specific type of microorganism), and should only be used when laboratory tests have confirmed that trichomonads are the cause of the infection. The antibacterial agent in FLAGYL, *metronidazole,* has been shown to be carcinogenic (cancer-causing) in mice and rats, and can destroy white blood cells (dangerously so with extended use).

People with liver diseases metabolize the drug slowly, which can result in a dangerous buildup of the drug in the blood. And anyone with a blood disorder should be monitored carefully by a doctor before and after therapy with FLAGYL. The drug is not recommended for pregnant women, since it crosses the placental barrier and can enter the fetal circulation rapidly. It's also unsafe to use in conjunction with anticoagulants since it potentiates the blood-thinning effects of these drugs. (If you're on anticoagulants, be sure your doctor knows that your gynecologist has prescribed FLAGYL because you'll probably need a prescription change during the course of *metronidazole* treatment.)

Side effects of nausea, headaches, diarrhea, and cramping are not uncommon, but these reactions can become quite severe if alcohol is consumed in conjunction with the drug. The drug has also been known to cause increased urination, loss of sexual desire, and incontinence.

Yes, there are a lot of risks involved in taking FLAGYL, but if it's prescribed, taken and monitored correctly, it's no more unsafe than hundreds of other medications.

CHAPTER XV

The Not-So-Miraculous Drugs

105. Think twice before taking these medicines

All that glitters isn't gold, and all the medications that doctors prescribe and pharmacies sell aren't the wonder-workers they've been cracked up to be.

The following is a list of medications that have been found to lack substantial evidence of effectiveness by the FDA's Drug Efficacy Study Implementation program.

(NOTE: These drugs have been deemed ineffective only in the dosage forms indicated.)

BRAND NAME	DOSAGE FORM	MANUFACTURER
ACTIFED-C EXPECTORANT	elixir	Burroughs Wellcome Co.
ADRENOSEM SALICYLATE	tablet; solution intramuscular	Beecham Labs
ALEVAIRE	inhalant solution	Breon; Winthrop
AMESEC	enteric coated tablet; capsule	Lilly

BRAND NAME	DOSAGE FORM	MANUFACTURER
AMINOPHYLLINE & AMYTAL	capsule	Lilly
ANANASE	enteric coated tablet	Rorer
ARLIDIN	tablet	USV
AVAZYME	enteric coated tablet	Wallace
AZO GANTANOL	tablet	Roche
BENTYL/ PHENOBARBI- TAL (does not apply to syrup)	capsule; tablet	Merrell Dow Pharmaceuticals
BETADINE VAGINAL GEL	gel	Purdue Frederick
BUTAZOLIDIN ALKA	tablet	Geigy
CANTIL w/ PHENOBARBI- TAL	tablet	Merrell Dow Pharmaceuticals
CALDECORT	ointment	Pennwalt
CARBRITAL	capsule; elixir	Parke-Davis
CARTRAX	tablet	Roerig
CELESTONE w/NEOMYCIN	cream	Schering
CETACAINE	aerosol; ointment; gel; liquid	Cetylite
CHYMORAL	enteric coated tablet	Armour Pharm.
COMBID	sustained release capsule	SKF

BRAND NAME	DOSAGE FORM	MANUFACTURER
CORDRAN-N	ointment; cream; lotion	Lilly
COROVAS	sustained release capsule	Amfre-Grant
CORTISPORIN	cream	Burroughs-Well-come
CYCLANDELATE	tablet	Cord Premo
CYCLOSPASMOL	capsule; tablet	Ives
DAINITE	tablet	Wallace
DAINITE-KL	tablet	Wallace
DARICON PB	tablet	Beecham Labs
DEANER	tablet	Riker
DEPROL	tablet	Wallace
DI-ADEMIL-K	tablet	Squibb
DIBENZYLINE (does not apply for treatment of pheochromo-cytoma)	capsule	SKF
DIUTENSEN	tablet	Wallace
DONNATAL EXTENTABS (applies only to controlled release product)	sustained release tablet	Robins
EQUAGESIC	tablet	Wyeth
EQUANITRATE	tablet	Wyeth
ERYTHROCIN	ointment	Abbott
ERYTHROMYCIN	ointment	Upjohn

BRAND NAME	DOSAGE FORM	MANUFACTURER
FLORINEF	lotion	Squibb
IODOCHLORHY-DROXYQUIN w/ HYDROCORTI-SONE	cream	Byk-Gulden
ISORDIL w/ PHENOBARBI-TAL	tablet	Ives
ISOXSUPRINE HCL	tablet	Cord Premo
KENALOG-S	ointment; cream; lotion	Squibb
LIBRAX	capsule	Roche
LUFYLLIN-EPG	tablet; elixir	Wallace
LUFTODIL	tablet	Wallace
MARAX	tablet; syrup	Roerig
MEPERGAN FORTIS	capsule	Wyeth
METI-DERM w/ NEOMYCIN	ointment; aerosol	Schering
MIDRIN	capsule	Reed & Carnrick
MIGRAL	tablet	Burroughs Well-come
MILPATH	tablet	Wallace
MILTRATE	tablet	Wallace
MYCO TRIACET	ointment	Premo
MYCOLOG	ointment; cream	Squibb
NATURETIN w/K	tablet	Squibb

BRAND NAME	DOSAGE FORM	MANUFACTURER
NEO-CORT-DOME	lotion; cream	Dome
NEO-CORTEF	ointment; lotion; cream	Upjohn
NEO-DELTA-CORTEF	ointment; lotion	Upjohn
NEO-HYDELTRASOL	lotion; ointment	Merck Sharp & Dohme
NEO-HYTONE	cream	Dermik Labs
NEO-MEDROL ACETATE	cream	Upjohn
NEO-NYSTA-CORT	ointment	Miles
NEO-OXYLONE	ointment	Upjohn
NEO-SYNALAR	cream	Syntex
NEODECADRON	cream	Merck Sharp & Dohme
NEOMYCIN SULFATE-HYDROCORTA-MATE HYDROCHLOR-IDE	ointment	Ulmer Pharmacal
NEOMYCIN SULFATE-HYDROCORTI-SONE	ointment	Premo Doak Pharmacal Ferndale Labs
NEOMYCIN SULFATE-HYDROCORTI-SONE ACETATE	ointment	American Pharmaceutical Biocraft Labs
NEOSPORIN	lotion	Burroughs Wellcome

BRAND NAME	DOSAGE FORM	MANUFACTURER
NEOSPORIN-G	cream	Burroughs Wellcome
NYLIDRIN HCL	tablet	Cord
NYSTAFORM-HC	ointment; lotion	Miles
NYSTATIN-NEOMYCIN SULFATE-GRAMICIDIN-TRIAMCINOLONE ACETONIDE	cream	Premo
ORENZYME	enteric coated tablet	Merrell Dow Pharmaceuticals
OXAINE M	suspension	Wyeth
PAPASE	chewable tablet	Warner-Lambert Parke-Davis
PATHIBAMATE	tablet	Lederle
PATHILON SEQUELS (doesn't apply to conventional dosage forms)	sustained release capsule	Lederle
PATHILON/ PHENOBARBITAL	tablet; sustained release capsule	Lederle
PERITRATE w/ PHENOBARBITAL	sustained release capsule; tablet	Warner-Lambert Parke-Davis
All pentylenetetrazol-containing products		

BRAND NAME	DOSAGE FORM	MANUFACTURER
POTABA	tablet, capsule; powder	Glenwood
PRISCOLINE	solution injectable	Ciba
PRO-BANTHINE w/ PHENOBAR-BITAL	tablet	Searle
QUADRINAL	tablet	Knoll
QUIBRON PLUS	capsule; elixir	Mead Johnson
RACET	cream	Lemmon Pharmacal
RAUTRAX	tablet	Squibb
RAUTRAX IMPROVED	tablet	Squibb
RAUTRAX-N	tablet	Squibb
RAUTRAX-N MODIFIED	tablet	Squibb
RONIACOL	tablet; sustained release tablet elixir	Roche
RUHEXATAL PB	tablet	Lemmon
RUHEXATAL & RESERPINE	tablet	Lemmon
SUPERTAH H-C	ointment	Purdue Frederick
SYNALGOS	capsule	Ives
SYNALGOS DC	capsule	Ives
TERRA-CORTRIL	ointment	Pfizer
TERRA-CORTRIL	aerosol	Pfizer
TIGAN (does not apply to capsules in 200 mg. or 400 mg. strengths)	capsule, suppository	Beecham

BRAND NAME	DOSAGE FORM	MANUFACTURER
TROCINATE	tablet	Poythress
VALPIN PB	tablet	Endo
VASOCON-A	solution	Cooper
VASODILAN	tablet; solution intramuscular	Mead Johnson
VIOFORM-HYDROCOR-TISONE	cream, ointment	Ciba
VYTONE	cream	Dermik Labs
WYANOIDS HC	suppository	Wyeth
ZACTANE	tablet	Wyeth
ZACTIRIN	tablet	Wyeth
ZACTIRIN COM-POUND 100	tablet	Wyeth

106. How good is your mouthwash?

If it's "antiseptic" it's not terrific, according to recommendations made recently by a Food and Drug Administration expert advisory committee.

According to the committee, antibacterial agents are not necessary to freshen the mouth. Also, aside from being unnecessary (that "clean breath" comes from the flavorings in the mouthwash and the act of rinsing the mouth itself), there's no evidence that those "germ-killing" agents are effective. In fact, they might even retard healing!

My advice is brush and floss regularly and try a simple supplement regimen of 1 chlorophyll tablet or capsule, 3 acidophilus capsules, and 50 mg. of zinc, all 1 to 3 times daily.

CAUTION: It's advised that mouthwashes which contain benzocaine or other pain relievers for relief of sore throats should not be used for more than 2 days or given to children under three years of age unless directed by a physician.

107. Any questions about Chapter XV?

I've read that several antibacterial topical ointments have been found ineffective and even dangerous for treating skin wounds. Are there any natural healing ointments for, let's say, burns or acne sores?

One of the best that I know is the Aloe Vera plant. This natural healer contains a substance called Aloe Vera Gel, which is a mixture of antibiotic, astringent, and coagulating agents, a pain inhibitor and a growth stimulator (also called a "wound hormone"), which accelerates the healing of injured surfaces. It's an immediate and effective aid for burns of any sort (as well as for acne, insect stings, and poison ivy), and it does not cause blisters or scars. Just split a leaf and apply the pulp directly to the wounded area or soak a small piece of cloth with the Aloe Vera Gel, and then bind it on. Vitamin E, 1,000 IU, used topically, can also help scarring from burns.

Someone told me that a cough medicine which combines an expectorant with a suppressant is ineffective. Is this true?

No, not necessarily, though some expectorant-suppressants have been deemed less than effective by the FDA. A cough suppressant, an antitussive, acts on the brain to suppress the cough reflex. An expectorant, such as the widely used *guaifenesin,* does not work on the brain but on the upper respiratory tract, thinning the thickness of bronchial secretions and thereby making it easier to cough up phlegm. They do not conflict. ROBITUSSIN-DM combines *dextromethorphan,* an effective cough suppressant that—unlike *codeine* or *hydrocodone* (suppressants often in prescription cough medicines)—has few side effects and a very low potential for abuse or dependence, and *guaifenesin,* an expectorant. Though there have been controversies about combination cough medicines, these two ingredients appear to have proved themselves effective in combination. My feeling is that when you begin adding other ingredients, such as an unnecessary decongestant, or an ingredient like *ammonium chloride* (an expectorant) which can be dangerous to people with lung, liver, or kidney problems, then you have trouble.

Part Five

SPECIAL FOR SENIOR CITIZENS

Chapter XVI

A Hard Look at the Golden Years

108. Why doctors prescribe too much, too often

As we grow older so do our bodies, and as happens with even the best machinery, age takes its toll and things can go wrong. But in this era of overabundant medication, far too many senior citizens are being given drugs not only for illnesses, but for *side effects* of drugs that they're already taking—side effects which mimic other conditions and are only compounded by the new side effect or interaction of yet another prescription drug.

109. How your age affects your medication

The physiological changes that occur with the aging process can alter the pharmacological properties of medicines in a number of ways.

1. *Absorption.* Because your gastrointestinal motility decreases with age, there is a slower emptying of the stomach and an increasing danger of two or more medicines remaining to interact adversely.
2. *Distribution.* Albumin, a protein in the bloodstream that tends to bind to many drugs, thereby limiting or inacti-

vating them, decreases in concentration as we age. Because of this, some drugs which were formerly controlled, or kept in check by albumin, become almost entirely unbound. This can cause you to develop an adverse reaction to a medication you've been taking for years, as well as make you more vulnerable to new drug interactions.

3. *Metabolism.* The ability of the liver to metabolize drugs also decreases with passing years. (Drinkers over forty are often surprised by their inability to "keep up with the boys" at cocktail time.) Because of this, drugs remain in your system longer, increasing the danger of serious drug interaction.

4. *Excretion.* Your kidneys are not immune to aging, and though they might function sufficiently to eliminate body wastes, their ability to excrete drugs does decrease. This, once again, can result in drug buildup and the possibility of adverse drug interactions.

110. Drug interactions for senior citizens to be aware of

IF YOU ARE TAKING . . .

ANTACIDS
(Alka-Seltzer, Gelusil, Maalox, Mylanta, Rolaids, Tums, etc.)

BE SURE YOU KNOW THAT . . .

- they can inhibit the absorption of *phenothiazine* tranquilizers (COMPAZINE, STELAZINE, THORAZINE, etc.) and the medications should not be taken within an hour of each other.

- if you take GERITOL or any other iron supplement, antacids containing *carbonate* or *magnesium trisilicate* (CHOOZ, GELUSIL, TUMS, etc.) can inhibit the iron absorption and therefore should be taken several hours apart.

- they increase the elimination of *aspirin* while slowing down its rate of absorption, therefore substantially reducing its levels of effectiveness.

- they can significantly decrease the absorption of LANOXIN and other *digitalis* medicines used to improve the efficiency of the heart (CEDILANID-D, DIGIFORTIS, CRY-STODIGIN, GITALIGIN, etc.), and therefore, should not be taken without consulting your doctor.

- some antacids (ALKA-SELTZER, ROLAIDS, TUMS) can increase the effectiveness of the heart rhythm drug *quinidine* (CARDIOQUIN, CINQUIN, DURAQUIN, QUINORA) to a dangerously unwanted degree, while others, such as AMPHO-JEL, can inhibit *quinidine's* effectiveness. Consult your doctor before taking *any* antacid.

- they can reduce the effectiveness of *tetracycline* antibiotics. (ROLAIDS might spell relief under some circumstances, but not these!)

- the beta-blocker INDERAL will be less effective if taken with antacids that contain *aluminum hydroxide* (AMPHOJEL, GELU-SIL, MAALOX, MYLANTA, etc.).

IF YOU ARE TAKING . . .

ASPIRIN
(Alka-Seltzer, Anacin, Bufferin, Dristan, Excedrin, Midol, Vanquish, etc.)

BE SURE YOU KNOW THAT . . .

- hundreds of OTC and prescription medicines contain *aspirin*.

- combining *aspirin* and any anticoagulant (see section 34) can be deadly.

- it can, ironically, diminish the effectiveness of prescription arthritis drugs (see section 41).

- it can potentiate diabetes drugs (see section 36) and lower blood sugar levels too much.

- it can be deadly if combined with the antimetabolite *methotrexate* (MEXATE), which is often used in the treatment of cancer.

- it can inhibit the effectiveness of antigout medications (see section 44).

- the analgesic properties of *aspirin* are diminished if you are also taking a diuretic containing *reserpine* (see section 40).

IF YOU ARE TAKING . . .

OTC COLD REMEDIES AND DECONGESTANTS
(Alka-Seltzer Plus, Allerest, Contac, Coricidin-D, Dristan, Neo-synephrine, Robitussin PE, Triaminic, etc.)

BE SURE YOU KNOW THAT . . .

- if you're taking an antidepressant (see section 35), these medications can raise your blood pressure to a lethally dangerous degree.

- with an antihypertensive medication (see section 40), these OTC products can either inhibit or potentiate the effectiveness. Be sure to check out *all* medications with your doctor!

- if you're taking any cortisone-like medication for asthma (HEXADROL, HYDROCORTONE, MEDROL, ORASONE, STERAPRED, KENALOG, etc.), the use of any OTC asthma medication may alter heart rhythms lethally!

- these medications can cause irregular heart function if taken in conjunction with such heart medicines as *digoxin* (LANOXIN).

- lethal interactions can occur if taken with *phenothiazines* (COMPAZINE, THORAZINE, STELAZINE, MELLARIL, etc.), the major tranquilizers, and any MAO inhibitor.

- headache medications containing *ergotamine* (BELLERGAL, CAFERGOT, CAFERMINE, ERGOMAR, ERGOSTAT, GYN-ERGEN, etc.) or drugs containing *belladonna and phenobarbital* (BELAP, CHARDONNA, OXOIDS, PHEN-O-BEL, etc.) can interact adversely with OTC cold remedies and decongestants and cause serious elevation of blood pressure.

IF YOU ARE TAKING . . .

LANOXIN (*digoxin*)

BE SURE YOU KNOW THAT . . .

- antacids can significantly decrease the absorption of the drug.

- *digoxin* should be taken at least one hour apart from other drugs.

- if taken with diuretics, you have an increased risk of digitalis toxicity.

- decreasing kidney function might mean you need a lower dosage of this medicine.

- if taking *quinidine* (CARDIOQUIN, DURAQUIN, QUINDRA) with this medicine, your serum level of *digoxin* is elevated, and you might need a lower dosage; frequent checks with your physician are recommended.

- laxatives, depending on which one you use, can either increase or decrease the effectiveness of *digoxin*.

IF YOU ARE TAKING . . .

LASIX (*furosemide*)
HYDRO DIURIL (*hydrochlorothiazide*)

BE SURE YOU KNOW THAT . . .

- taking these drugs with a digitalis medicine increases the risk of digitalis toxicity because of low potassium levels.

- potassium levels can be altered by decreased kidney function and supplements might *not* be needed.

IF YOU ARE TAKING . . .

COUMADIN (*warfarin sodium*)
PANWARFIN (*warfarin sodium*)
ATHROMBIN-K (*warfarin potassium*)

BE SURE YOU KNOW THAT . . .

- taking any medication that contains *aspirin* with these drugs can cause severe bleeding and can be deadly.

- these medications, taken in combination with such urinary-tract anti-infectives as BACTRIM or SEPTRA can result in *warfarin* toxicity or severe bleeding.

- thyroid medications, such as PROLOID, SYNTHROID, etc., can increase the blood-thinning effectiveness of *warfarin* to a potentially dangerous degree.

- the antiarthritic drug INDOCIN (*indomethacin*) can interact adversely with *warfarin*, causing hemorrhage, and without proper monitoring the combination could be deadly.

- DORIDEN (*glutethimide*), often used to treat insomnia, can seriously decrease the effectiveness of *warfarin*, as can many other sedatives and tranquilizers. Be sure to check with your doctor before taking *any* other medication if you're on anticoagulants. (See section 34.)

111. Why seniors need senior nutrition

Senior citizens consume more drugs than any other age group. Chronic diseases of older people, such as hypertension, heart disease, congestive heart failure, peripheral vascular disease, bronchitis, emphysema, arthritis, cancer, and many others, all lend themselves to single or multiple drug prescriptions—and these drugs take their toll nutritionally. In fact, many senior citizens from all economic brackets suffer from subclinical nutritional deficiencies because of marginal intakes of key nutrients due to malabsorption, poor teeth, depression, loneliness and other social problems.

MOST COMMON NUTRIENT DEFICIENCIES

Folic acid	(caused by such drugs as MEXATE, QUESTRAN, DILANTIN, and others, along with low intakes of fresh fruits and green vegetables)
Calcium	(caused by such drugs as *phenobarbital*, DECADRON, HALDRONE, HEXADROL, and other glucocorticoids, as well as all diuretics and an insufficient intake of dairy products)
Vitamin B_{12}	(caused by drugs such as *colchicine* and QUESTRAN, as well as insufficient intakes of liver, milk, eggs, and cheese)
Vitamin D	(caused by use of drugs such as DILANTIN and insufficient amounts of sunlight)

As a general rule, if you're over 65 you need extra minerals (especially calcium, magnesium, and iron) and extra vitamins E, C, and B as well. (See section 55.)

112. A super simple supplement regimen for seniors

Twice a day with breakfast and dinner take a multiple vitamin and mineral; rose hips vitamin C, 500 mg. (with bioflavonoids); a multiple chelated mineral tablet; and vitamin E, 200–400 IU (dry form).

113. Retarding the aging process naturally

Our bodies are made up of millions of cells, each with a life of around two years or less. But before a cell dies it reproduces itself, though with some alteration (which is why we don't look exactly as we did ten years ago). Unfortunately this alteration is basically deterioration. In short, as our cells change and deteriorate, we grow old.

> Growing old doesn't have to mean wrinkles!

But growing old doesn't have to mean wrinkles or spotted and brittle skin. There is a way you can look and feel six to twelve years younger, and it has nothing to do with cosmetic surgery or the fountain of youth—it's nucleic acids!

Dr. Benjamin S. Frank, author of *Nucleic Acid Therapy in Aging and Degenerative Disease* (New York: Psychological Library, 1969; revised 1974), has found that deteriorating cells can be rejuvenated if provided with substances that directly nourish them. These substances are nucleic acids.

RNA (ribonucleic acid) and DNA (deoxyribonucleic acid) are the nucleic acids in our bodies. DNA, essentially a chemical boiler plate for new cells, sends out RNA molecules to form them. When the boss, DNA, stops giving orders to RNA, cell construction stops—as does life.

According to Dr. Frank, we need 1 to 1½ grams of nucleic

acids daily. Though we produce our own, they're broken down too quickly to help retard the aging process, so they must be supplied from external sources.

BEST SOURCES OF NUCLEIC ACIDS

Wheat germ, bran, spinach, asparagus, mushrooms, fish (especially sardines, salmon, and anchovies), chicken liver, oatmeal, onions, beans, and nutritional yeast

FOR OPTIMUM RESULTS

- Fish should be eaten 7 times weekly.
- Skim milk (two 8 oz. glasses) daily
- Fruit or vegetable juice (one 8 oz. glass daily)
- Water (preferably spring) (four 8 oz. glasses daily) (The large fluid intake is vital, because a high RNA diet may also raise your uric acid level.)

114. Mindell RNA-DNA "YOUNGER THAN SPRINGTIME" supplement regimen

- RNA-DNA 100 mg. tablets (one daily for one month, then 2 daily for the next month, then 3 daily thereafter for 6 days each week)
- High-potency multiple vitamin with chelated minerals (time-release preferred)
- Vitamin C, 1,000 mg.
- Vitamin E (dry form) 200–400 IU
- Stress B-complex
      All taken A.M. and P.M. with meals.

115. Another route to retard aging: S.O.D.

S.O.D. (Super Oxide Dismutase) is an enzyme, manufactured by the body, that fights off cell-deteriorating agents and prevents them from attacking cells.

It's possible that you can increase your life span!

As we grow older, the S.O.D. levels in our bodies are reduced, and the cell attackers, called free radicals, begin their ruthless war on collagen (the "cement" that holds cells together), causing it to become inflexible and accelerating the aging process, which is evidenced by wrinkles and stiffening of limbs.

Supplements of S.O.D., which are available in 125 mcg. tablets, taken daily for six days a week, can fortify the body against the ravages of free radicals. No guarantees of perpetual youth can be given, but S.O.D. has been cited in major medical journals as a substance that can possibly "increase the average life span by 5 or more years."

116. Laxatives are not the cure-all for hemorrhoids

Laxatives (see section 48) are the most abused drug by the elderly. Because of the decreased gastrointestinal motility that occurs with aging, many older people get into the "Laxative Habit," which usually causes rebound constipation, straining at stool, and hemorrhoids (piles), which are often the reason laxatives have been taken to begin with.

Hemorrhoids are irregular or tortuous swellings of the veins under the lining of the anus and lower rectum. *Internal hemorrhoids* are covered by the mucous membrane; *external hemorrhoids* are just beneath the skin. The swellings become more prominent when you strain at stool. Under this stress the hemorrhoids can enlarge quite suddenly and fill with blood clots. These clots are usually quite painful and may break down and bleed profusely for several days.

117. How to handle a hemorrhoid—naturally

Keeping your stool soft is important to prevent the straining which increases hemorrhoidal swelling. One tablespoon of unprocessed bran three times a day can help, along with vitamin C, 1,000 mg. 2 to 4 times a day (make sure the vitamin C contains bioflavonoids!). The vitamin C keeps the stool soft and strengthens the walls of the blood vessels.

Vitamin E, which can help to prevent and dissolve blood clots, alleviates the clots which make hemorrhoids so painful. I'd recommend 200–400 IU 1 to 3 times daily, along with vitamin E concentrated oil, which, when applied locally to the affected area, reduces discomfort.

Steer clear of coffee, chocolate, cocoa, and cola; these have been known to increase anal itching. Also, learn to lift objects by stooping instead of bending. In this way, you reduce the abdominal pressure on hemorrhoidal veins.

118. Any questions about Chapter XVI?

My father, who's 85, lives with us and suffers from heartburn. He's taking so many medicines already, I'm reluctant to offer him even an OTC antacid. Is there any sort of "natural" way I can help him?

Prevention is the best natural medicine. I'd suggest that you monitor his diet and keep him away from any fried and spicy foods, chocolate, processed luncheon meats, as well as alcohol and coffee. You'll be surprised how these basic restrictions can help.

If he does get an attack of heartburn, *don't* have him lie down after eating, *do* make sure his clothes aren't fitted too tightly around his waist, and when he does go to sleep, keep the head of his bed raised about six inches (you can do this by putting blocks under the legs at the top of his bed).

Is there a government agency that handles health problems of senior citizens?

The National Institute on Aging, Building 31, Room 5C35, Bethesda, Md. 20205. They have an enormous amount of free information available on senior citizen health problems.

My father, who's 74, is upset when his doctor refuses to give him antibiotics when he (my dad) is convinced that he needs them. Does the doctor have reasons we don't know about for not prescribing antibiotics?

I'm sure that he does. In the first place, the reduced functioning of liver cells in senior citizens makes it difficult for them to detoxify antibiotics, which could result in hepatoxicity (liver poisoning). In the second place, older people are more susceptible to the effects of rapid heartbeat and sodium in some antibiotics. Also, according to Dr. Joel D. Posner, who has studied the effects of antibiotics on elderly persons, the attack of antibiotics on the diminished alveolar units in lungs of aging persons can cause unwanted complications. Additionally, the lessened kidney function of older persons makes it difficult for them to eliminate antibiotics, which could lead to higher than wanted serum levels of the drugs. And if that's not enough, there's the fact that *sodium penicillin* can cause sodium-retention and congestive heart failure. Also, senior citizens are usually more susceptible to antibiotic-caused diarrhea and colitis. My advice is that your father should listen to his doctor.

CHAPTER XVII

Arthritis

119. What it is

Arthritis is basically an inflammation of a joint or joints, and there are many forms and causes of the disease.

- It can strike persons of any age.
- It can be caused by an injury as well as a complication of another disease (e.g., rubella).
- It can exist as a symptom accompanying a systemic infection.
- It can occur as a side effect of certain medications—particularly anticonvulsants, contraceptives, and major tranquilizers.
- Osteoarthritis and rheumatoid arthritis are only two of the approximately one hundred conditions known as rheumatic diseases.
- Rheumatic diseases encompass tendinitis, hepatitis, gout, syphilis, diabetes mellitus, multiple myeloma, and more.

120. Arthritis drugs—pro and con

Advantages   *Disadvantages*

ASPIRIN

least toxic anti-inflammatory drug

causes gastric bleeding

can cause ringing in the ears and/or reversible deafness with high doses that are necessary for arthritis treatment

can interact adversely with other drugs commonly taken for arthritis, such as INDOCIN, increasing risk of stomach ulceration and bleeding

NONASPIRIN SALICYLATES (MAGAN, TRILISATE, DISALCID)

cause less gastric bleeding because they dissolve in gastric fluids quickly

insufficient data on whether they are as effective as *aspirin*

NONSTEROIDAL ANTI-INFLAMMATORIES (NALFON, MOTRIN, NAPROSYN, CLINORIL, and TOLECTIN)

most are equivalent to *aspirin* in effectiveness

generally cause less gastrointestinal distress

CLINORIL can cause the same adverse effects as INDOCIN, such as congestive heart failure

all nonsteroidal drugs can cause salt retention, which can lead to congestive heart failure (CLINORIL and INDOCIN are just more potent than most of the other drugs)

may cause light-headedness and hallucinations in older people

MOTRIN, NALFON, and NAPROSYN can cause serious kidney toxicity

may have side effects that are as yet unknown

the safety of CLINORIL for long-term use has not been established

INDOCIN

very effective in treating osteoarthritis of the hip

can aid in treatment of tendinitis, bursitis, and other musculoskeletal disorders

can cause gastric ulceration

can cause congestive heart failure

because it can reduce fever and inflammation, it can mask signs of an infection leading to a dangerous delay in treatment

GOLD INJECTIONS

can cause permanent remissions in early rheumatoid arthritis

can temporarily stop disease progress in joints and relieve morning stiffness

can cause such serious side effects as kidney disease and bone marrow depression

adversely affects the skin and mucous membranes of the mouth

(Gold compounds are only used to treat rheumatoid arthritis that progresses despite adequate regimens of *aspirin*, rest, and physical therapy.)

CORTISONE

can only relieve symptoms

increases susceptibility to infection

can cause fluid retention, gastrointestinal problems, unwanted facial hair, mental depression, facial puffiness, and lead to osteoporosis

121. Diet can help

Though conclusive evidence is not yet in, there are enough established correlations between arthritic disease and nutrition to make you pay a lot more attention to what you should and shouldn't eat.

For example, arthritis is a collagen disease, and vitamin C is necessary for the formation of normal collagen fiber. Gout, another form of arthritis, is related to an excess of uric acid, meaning foods that cause an increase in uric acid (such as beans, peas, liver, and others high in purine) should be avoided. (See section 125.)

SOME ARTHRITIS DIET TIPS

- Avoid coffee, tea, soft drinks, sugar, alcohol, and all refined carbohydrates.
- Increase your intake of vegetables (see section 122 for how to get the most vitamins from them).
- Eat more raw vegetables.
- Exclude foods in the nightshade family of vegetables, which include—among others—potatoes, tomatoes, and eggplant.

- Increase your intake of vitamin-C-rich foods (see section 55).
- Take the right supplements!

I recommend the following regimen:

High-potency multiple vitamin with chelated minerals (time-release preferred)	A.M. & P.M.
High-potency chelated multiple minerals	A.M. & P.M.
Vitamin C	1,000 mg, 1 to 3 times daily (if you're taking a lot of *aspirin,* you're losing a *lot* of vitamin C)
Vitamin B-complex	100 mg. 1 to 3 times daily
Vitamin B$_{12}$	100–2,000 mcg. daily
Niacin	50–1,000 mg. (that's the ceiling) daily
Yucca tabs	1 to 3, 3 times daily
Pantothenic acid	100 mg. 3 times daily
Vitamin A and Vitamin D	10,000 IU 400 IU } 3 times daily (take for 5 days and stop for 2)
OR Cod liver oil	1 to 2 tbsp. 3 times daily (if capsules, 3 caps 3 times daily) Again, take for 5 days and stop for 2.

122. How to hyper-vitaminize your foods

- Cut fruits and vegetables when you're ready to eat them. (Vitamins are lost when these foods are left standing.)
- Wash but don't soak fresh vegetables (you'll lose needed vitamins B and C).
- Don't thaw frozen vegetables before cooking.
- Cook vegetables quickly in smallest amount of water. (Microwaving keeps more vitamins in.)
- Use converted and parboiled rice instead of polished rice. (Brown rice is more nutrient-rich than white.)

- Cooking in iron pots can give you the benefit of that mineral, but can shortchange you on vitamin C.
- Don't use baking soda when cooking vegetables. (It destroys thiamine and vitamin C.)
- Cook potatoes in their skins.
- Copper pots are pretty but can destroy vitamin C, folic acid, and vitamin E.

123. Exercise is essential

Exercise can relieve pain, strengthen endurance, increase muscle tone, counteract anxiety, and prevent arthritic conditions from worsening, but there is disagreement on what sort and when exercise should be instituted.

Most of the disagreement comes from the fact that inflammation is reduced by rest, but too much rest will cause tendons to weaken and bones to soften. But there are physiatrists—MDs who specialize in physical medicine and rehabilitation—and these doctors can design a personalized exercise program that would be right for your needs. Your best bet would be to check with your local Arthritis Foundation for a recommendation of a doctor in your area.

After consulting with a physician, try to find ways to incorporate exercise into your daily routine. As a general rule, avoid exercise that burdens weight-bearing joints (sports such as tennis or jogging), and apply your energies to activities such as yoga or swimming.

Keep your weight down to avoid unnecessary stress on weight-bearing joints.

124. Fight arthritis with sex

One of the best ways to ease arthritic pain, according to recent research, is to keep up a regular sex life.

> Sex gives patients from 4 to 6 hours of relief from arthritis pain.

Sex can act as an analgesic through adrenal stimulation. According to Dr. Jessie E. Potter, director of the National Institute for Human Relationships, in a speech given at the National Arthritis Foundation symposium, "Sex gives patients from four to six hours of relief from arthritis pain, probably by stimulating increased production of cortisone."

Sex as a pain reliever, by the way, doesn't necessarily mean intercourse. According to Dr. Potter, any kind of sexual arousal— self-stimulation, petting, oral sex—leads to cortisone release. In other words, though it might take two to tango, you don't need a partner to fight arthritis with sex.

125. Any questions about Chapter XVII?

My uncle used DMSO and said it helped his arthritis. He said it could be bought without prescription, but I can't find it anywhere. What is it and where can I get it?

DMSO (*dimethyl sulfoxide*) is essentially a by-product of the paper industry that has been used as an antifreeze, among other things. In the early 1960s it was found to be a good anti-inflammatory drug that could be applied topically. But the FDA found that the drug could rapidly enter the bloodstream and cause a loss of vision, along with nausea, skin rash, and other unpleasant side effects.

The drug is approved for veterinary use, but as far as humans are concerned, it's only approved for treatment of a rare bladder condition known as interstitial cystitis. The FDA is concerned about its unknown purity and quality, but desperate arthritis sufferers have been purchasing the product as a degreaser or an art supply through the mail. Essentially, it's an under-the-counter drug, and I'd recommend steering clear of it. There have been reports of skin and mucous membrane burns because of using the drug topically, and to date the FDA position is that "there is insufficient evidence to show that DMSO is either safe or effective in treating arthritis or bursitis." Your uncle might have been lucky; you might not be.

I've always used heat to alleviate my arthritis pain, but my friend told me that ice works better. Is this true?

Moist heat has always been a standard arthritis pain-reliever, but recent research at the Germantown Medical Center in Philadelphia has shown that wrapping the inflamed joint in ice packs can bring noticeable relief to sufferers of rheumatoid arthritis. In fact, after four weeks patients reported that they felt less pain, took fewer drugs, slept longer, and could move more easily.

Are there any foods that are particularly good for combatting arthritis?

Alfalfa sprouts top the list. Studies have shown that they're rich in the trace minerals that are in short supply in rheumatoid and osteo-arthritis sufferers. (These trace minerals include zinc, manganese, molybdenum, chromium, tin, and aluminum.)

Also, according to Dr. Donald A. Gerber, associate professor of medicine at Downstate Medical Center in New York, eating a lot of high-histidine foods, such as eggs, whole milk, liver, fish, wheat germ, soybean meal, brown rice, brewer's yeast, dried peas, beans, and soybeans can prevent or possibly relieve early symptoms of the disease.

What are the high purine foods that can trigger gout attacks?

Because gout is a metabolic disorder that results in inefficient processing of purines (which, when broken down, produce uric acid as a by-product), foods that are high in these substances are best avoided. Purines are found mainly in fatty meats (pork) and poultry (goose, duck); in certain fish and shellfish (scallops, anchovies, clams); in organ meats (liver, sweetbreads, kidneys); in vegetables such as spinach, lentils, mushrooms, peas, and asparagus as well as in condiments, rich pastries, fried foods, and alcohol.

Does drinking alcohol cause gout?

No, but it can worsen the condition or trigger a gout attack, primarily because alcohol can alter the metabolism.

CHAPTER XVIII

High Blood Pressure

126. How dangerous is it?

High blood pressure (hypertension) is one of the most dangerous diseases you can get. Each year an estimated 850,000 people die because of it. Very often symptomless, the disease can, if untreated, affect your brain, vision, heart, blood vessels, and kidneys.

> It's one of the most dangerous diseases to get—
> and one of the easiest to treat.

If you're one of the sixty million Americans who have high blood pressure and are between the ages of 45 and 74, your risk is three times greater for a heart attack and seven times greater for a stroke than people with normal blood pressure.

Ironically, it's one of the easiest diseases to detect and treat.

127. Heading for high blood pressure

You're more prone to hypertension if

- someone in your family has it
- you're overweight
- your intake of salty or cholesterol-packed foods is high
- you suffer from stress or anxiety
- you smoke

128. What's normal and what's "high"?

As a general rule, you're considered within the normal range if your higher (systolic) pressure falls between 100 and 140, and the lower (diastolic) pressure is in the range of 60 to 90. A reading of 120/80 is considered normal for a healthy young adult.

Most doctors consider your diastolic (lower) pressure the key indicator of hypertension. For instance, mild hypertension would be a diastolic reading from about 90–105; moderate hypertension from 105–120; severe from 120–140; and very severe for any diastolic reading above 140.

129. How to bring down what's gone up

Early diagnosis can give you a head start on the right track down. Regular medical checkups are best, but you can purchase a sphygmomanometer and easily learn to keep tabs on your own pressure.

WAYS DOWN

- Antihypertensive drugs (see section 40), which include diuretics, vasodilators, and beta-blockers among others, are effective if taken as directed, if side effects are expected and understood, and if all precautions for drug and/or food interactions are observed.
- Adequate rest.
- Regular exercise. (Dr. Robert Cade, professor of medicine at the University of Florida, has found that aerobic exercises such as running, brisk walking, and bike riding caused a significant drop in blood pressure for 96

percent of patients who tried it. Check with your physician on a regimen that's okay for you.)

- Yoga exercise, which produces mental and physical relaxation.
- Biofeedback and relaxation techniques.
- Learning to speak more slowly. (Research at the University of Maryland School of Medicine has shown that if you speak more slowly, pausing for adequate breaths of air, you can gradually lower your blood pressure naturally!)
- Diet.
  - a) reduce if overweight
  - b) keep to a low-salt diet (see section 130)
  - c) increase your intake of potassium-rich foods (see section 55) unless contraindicated by your medication
  - d) stay away from caffeine (chocolate, colas, coffee, tea, etc.)
  - e) reduce your sugar intake
  - f) avoid cholesterol-rich foods
  - g) eat more onions and garlic (onions contain prostaglandin A1, a hormone-like substance that can lower blood pressure, and garlic has been shown in recent tests to significantly lower blood pressure in hypertensives)
- Stop smoking.
- Avoid stress or anxiety-provoking situations. (Jangling everyday noises such as car engines, horns, even loud televisions can cause stress and elevate blood pressure.)

130. How to keep your salt intake down

- Don't eat cured meat, such as ham, bacon, corned beef, or frankfurters; sausage; shellfish; any canned or frozen meat, poultry, or fish to which sodium has been added.
- When dining out, ask for an inside cut of meat, or chops or steaks without added salt.
- Look for the words *SALT, SODIUM,* or the chemical symbol *Na* when reading food labels.

- Don't drink or cook with water treated by a home water-softener; it adds sodium to the water.
- Stay away from laxatives and antacids, most of which contain plenty of sodium.
- Avoid the use of baking soda, monosodium glutamate (MSG, Accent), and baking powder in food preparation.
- Watch out for fast-food burgers. A Big Mac has 963 mg. of sodium and a Burger King Whopper has a whopping *1,038 mg. of sodium!* (Avoid their shakes, too, which usually contain from 275 to 685 mg. of salt.)
- Be aware that canned food (especially soups) and frozen dinners are usually very high in sodium. Check those labels!

131. Cooking tips for salt lovers

Salt-free foods don't have to be bland; you can liven them up with herbs and spices.

For eggs, try dill, oregano, or chopped chives (alone or mixed together).

Oatmeal can still be tasty without salt if you add a dash of cinnamon, a tiny bit of ginger, and a bit of lemon peel.

Meat loaf can be just as scrumptious salt-free if you add chopped onions, tomatoes, and celery (including the tops).

Meat soups can do without salt if you add a bay leaf and some vinegar or lemon juice.

All roast meat can still retain plenty of flavor without salt if you try using garlic and onion powder along with a bay leaf.

As for mashed potatoes—first boil the potatoes with a clove of garlic and some fresh parsley. When mashing the potatoes, add additional chopped parsley, cayenne pepper, and paprika. (For an exotic touch you can try a bit of curry powder.)

132. Any questions about Chapter XVIII?

Can anyone get high blood pressure?
Yes, even children, although it's rare. Some people, though,

are more vulnerable than others. For example, despite the fact that hypertension affects both sexes at all ages, it's more likely for males to get it under 50 and females after 60. And blacks, whose incidence of hypertension is almost *twice* that of the rest of the population, are generally afflicted at an earlier age.

As you get older, do you develop high blood pressure?

Many people do, but according to a study undertaken by Dr. Lot Page of Tufts University, they don't have to. Dr. Page found that primitive people in the Solomon Islands, untouched by our "civilized" eating and living habits, did *not* develop high blood pressure with aging. In other words, just because the candles on your birthday cake increase, it doesn't mean your blood pressure has to.

Can high blood pressure cause unusual mood swings or depression?

Noticeable mood changes or depression are not caused by hypertension, but they can be caused by medications that are given to patients with hypertension. Usually, this is the result of drugs that cause the patient to lose too much potassium. The diuretic LASIX, for example, often prescribed for hypertensives, can cause major mood swings and depression because of depleting too much potassium. Before consulting a psychiatrist, ask your physician about dietary supplements or a change of medication.

I have high blood pressure. Is there any way to tell whether or not my child will get it?

According to a recent study from the Mayo Clinic in Rochester, Minnesota, there is. By immersing one arm in ice water and checking the blood pressure of the other, a process called the Cold Pressor Test, they can tell whether your child will suffer hypertension later in life. If the blood pressure in the dry arm soars, it's more than likely he or she will develop high blood pressure. This can be enormously helpful, since preventive measures can be taken early on to drastically reduce any risk of stroke or heart attack.

Are there any vitamin or mineral deficiencies that could cause high blood pressure?

It's a possibility. In a study conducted by Dr. David A. McCarron, a professor at the Oregon Health Sciences University in Portland, a small but significant percentage of hypertensives tested showed less ionized calcium in their blood.

Help for Your Heart

133. Hardhearted heart disease facts

Heart disease is still the number one killer of Americans. According to cardiologist James Schoenberger, professor of preventive medicine at Chicago's Rush-Presbyterian-St. Luke's Medical Center, the problem can't really be solved with beta or calcium blockers, heart transplants, coronary bypasses, or other forms of palliative medicine. But, says Dr. Schoenberger, the disease *is* largely preventable!

> Heart disease is America's number one killer— but it can be prevented!

Let's take a look at the facts:

- Men have a higher incidence of coronary-artery disease than premenopausal women.
- Diabetics have a greater risk of heart disease.
- Your risk of developing heart disease is greater if close family members have had heart attacks.

- Whites in the United States have more frequent heart attacks than Blacks or Orientals.
- Risk of heart attack increases with cigarette smoking, high cholesterol levels, high blood pressure, excess weight, tension, stress, physical inactivity, and age.

134. How to defend your heart from attacks

1. *Check your blood pressure regularly* (see sections 127 and 128).
2. *Decrease your consumption of sugar.* Sugar raises your serum cholesterol and triglycerides (blood fats) as well as insulin levels. Also, anyone who has trouble properly metabolizing carbohydrates can endanger their heart.
3. *Stop smoking.* The longer you stay away from cigarettes, the more your risk of coronary heart disease approaches that of people who've never smoked at all.
4. *Exercise regularly.* Vigorous, regular physical exercise not only decreases your risk of coronary heart disease, but releases brain chemicals called endorphines, which give you a feeling of well-being.
5. *Watch your weight.* Too many extra pounds can be lethal. The Framingham Study, among many others, has linked increased coronary mortality with obesity.
6. *Cut down on your salt consumption.* Whether it's sodium chloride (table salt), sodium nitrate, sodium nitrite, monosodium glutamate (MSG), or sodium bicarbonate, they all contain sodium, which has been linked to the development of high blood pressure. (See section 129.)
7. *Decrease your consumption of saturated fats, hydrogenated oils, and cholesterol.* Eat less meat, butter, cheese, cream, and whole milk. Try to increase your polyunsaturated oils, such as sunflower, safflower, corn, and soy. Also, make sure you buy the cold-pressed oils.
8. *Eat more fresh fruit.* Apples and many citrus fruits are not only nutritious and virtually fat-free, but contain pectin, a dietary fiber that can help lower serum cholesterol levels.

9. *Eat more garlic.* It can do more than keep away were-wolves. Studies have shown that raw garlic (as well as onions and carrots) can significantly reduce several forms of circulating cholesterol in the body. (Deodorized garlic capsules are available.)

10. *Squeeze more vitamin C into your diet.* A study in the February 1981 issue of *Journal of Human Nutrition* has shown that vitamin C deficiencies, especially in older people, appear to play a role in the development of coronary heart disease.

11. *Be sure you're getting enough calcium.* Calcium reduces serum cholesterol and triglycerides. Chelated calcium, 1,000–1,200 mg. is a worthwhile daily supplement.

12. *Switch to soy protein.* Soy protein, in place of animal protein, has been shown to produce a 14 percent decrease in serum cholesterol after 2 weeks and a 21 percent reduction after 3 weeks in patients with elevated cholesterol.

13. *Get enough vitamin E.* This versatile vitamin raises the level of the "good" high-density lipoprotein (HDL) cholesterol, while it lowers the "bad" very low-density lipoprotein (VLDL) cholesterol and triglycerides. It can also help keep platelets (tiny disk-shaped blood cells) from "clumping up" on arterial walls.

14. *Fill up on fish.* The essential fatty acids (EPA and DHA) found in salmon, mackerel, anchovies, and so on, help to reduce platelet clumping.

15. *Maximize your magnesium.* A deficiency of magnesium can cause brief spasms of the coronary arteries, which can trigger a heart attack. A sufficient amount of this mineral would be 500 mg. a day. (For natural foods high in magnesium, see section 55.)

16. *Supplement the lecithin in your diet.* Lecithin can enhance fat metabolism. It's available in capsules, tablets, granules, or liquid. (I'd recommend 3 tbsp. liquid daily or 3 capsules 3 times daily.)

17. *Make sure you're getting enough vitamin B6.* A deficiency of vitamin B_6 can cause the production of a harmful amino acid. This amino acid causes destruction of tis-

sues and, when combined with cholesterol, may be responsible for the increased blockage of arteries.

18. *Keep away from caffeine.* Aside from depleting your body of needed B vitamins, caffeine is considered a culprit in hypertensive heart disease. Also, according to a report in the British medical journal *Lancet,* people who drink five cups of coffee a day have a 50 percent greater chance of having heart attacks than noncoffee-drinkers.

19. *Learn to relax.* Try yoga, meditation, biofeedback, because stress and tension can increase your risk of heart attack.

20. *Laughter can be great medicine.* Laughter is a complex, physiological exercise involving biochemical, endocrine, and circulatory systems, which can work together, release pent-up emotions, and help protect against heart disease.

135. Diet tips to keep you young (and healthy) at heart

Use lean meats, fish, chicken, turkey, and veal more often than beef, lamb, pork, and ham (which contain more fat).

When buying hamburger, look for the medium-to-deep reddish color that signifies a low fat content (a light pink color is a pretty good indication that excess fat has been ground in with the meat). What's even better is to select a well-trimmed piece of beef and have the butcher grind that for you.

Stay away from organ meats such as brain, heart, liver, sweetbreads, giblets, and so on, because they're much higher in cholesterol than animal muscle meat.

Make sure the "vegetable oil" on a manufacturer's label is not one of the *saturated* oils (coconut oil, cocoa butter, palm oil, or hydrogenated vegetable fat).

Use *polyunsaturated* oils (corn, cottonseed, safflower, sesame seed, soybean, sunflower seed, and walnut). When reading labels, make sure they say polyunsaturated or *liquid* corn (cottonseed, safflower, etc.) oil.

When buying margarine, be sure that the first ingredient is *liquid* oil. Tub margarines tend to be more polyunsaturated than stick forms.

Use fat-free or low-fat dairy products.

Select cheeses that are high in protein but low in fat. Good choices would be farmer's cheese, dry cottage cheese, and pot cheese. (Cheeses made from partially skimmed milk—ricotta, mozzarella, parmesan—are okay in small amounts.)

Don't buy frozen or canned food mixtures that contain fat, since you can't tell what sort of fat or how much is actually in it.

If you're nuts about nuts, eat walnuts. They're the highest in polyunsaturated fat among commonly used nuts. (Avoid cashews, peanuts, and Brazil nuts; they have at least twice the saturated fat of other commonly used nuts.)

See section 39 for more tips.

136. To eat eggs or not to eat eggs, that's still the question

The answer for you will have to come from your doctor, but it's worth mentioning that though the egg consumption in the United States is one-half what it was in 1945, there has *not* been a comparable decline in heart disease.

Though the American Heart Association still feels that more than 3 egg yolks a week can be hazardous, members of the American Medical Association feel otherwise. New research has shown that cholesterol behaves differently depending on the protein to which it is bound. Lipoproteins are the factors in our blood which transport cholesterol. Very low-density lipoproteins (VLDL) do seem to bear a correlation to heart disease, but high-density lipoproteins (HDL), which are composed principally of lecithin whose detergent action breaks up cholesterol, appear to have the opposite effect. In other words, the higher your HDL, the lower your chances of developing symptoms of heart disease.

What, you might ask, has all this to do with eggs? Well, not only do eggs have the most perfect protein components of any food, but they contain lecithin—and they *raise* HDL levels!

137. Any questions about Chapter XIX?

Is there any special supplement program that you'd recommend for someone with a heart condition?

Anyone with a heart condition should be under a doctor's care, and even though many people have found the following regimen effective, it should be discussed with your physician first.

- High-potency multiple vitamin
  with chelated minerals (time-
  release preferred)   A.M. & P.M.
- Vitamin C   1,000 mg., A.M. & P.M.
- High-potency chelated
  multiple mineral   A.M. & P.M.
- Vitamin B   100 mg., A.M. & P.M.
- Vitamin E   400 IU (dry form) 1 daily
- Niacin   100 mg., 1 to 3 times daily
- Lecithin   3 capsules or 1 tbsp. granules
                                        3 times daily

CHAPTER XX

Diabetes

138. Special problems for the elderly

The object of diabetes treatment is to restore a proper carbohydrate balance in the system while maintaining a good nutritional status. Because the disease occurs when the body is unable to fully metabolize sugars and starches (either because the pancreas doesn't produce enough insulin for processing, or the insulin produced is less than effective), medication and/or diet regulation is required.

Diabetics, generally prone to atherosclerosis and other complications, unfortunately face additional problems when they become senior citizens, mainly because they're usually on additional medications—and they're not properly alerted to the potential adverse interactions.

139. Drugs that can increase or decrease your blood sugar— too much!

If you're taking antidiabetic medication, check with your doctor, as well as with section 36 in this book, and make sure you know what can happen to your blood sugar when you mix medicines.

Aspirin, for example, can lower your blood sugar too far, as can the beta-blocker INDERAL. Thyroid medication, on the other hand, can elevate blood sugar levels and necessitate an increase in your present drug dosage.

Be particularly aware of the arthritis medicine *phenylbutazone* (BUTAZOLIDIN), which in combination with an oral antidiabetic drug can be dangerous in older people.

140. What you should know about testing your urine for sugar

Over-the-counter home testing products such as TES-TAPE, DIASTIX, and CLINISTIX are safe, simple, and fairly reliable if the manufacturer's instructions (as well as your doctor's) are followed exactly.

Because every individual has a different capacity to see the various shades of red, violet, blue, green, and so on, I'd advise consulting your pharmacist or physician on the best glucose home test for you. (TES-TAPE estimates glucose by grading shades of green; CLINISTIX by red to purple, and DIASTIX by blue to brown.)

141. A guide for testing urine

- A midstream sample of your first morning urine is best.
- Sample should be collected in a clean, dry container that has no detergent or chemical residue which could chemically interfere with test results.
- Test should be done as soon as possible after voiding, because room temperatures can change urine chemistry rapidly.
- Never freeze a urine specimen, though you can refrigerate it for a few hours if necessary. (Before testing, though, be sure specimen has been at room temperature for at least 15 minutes; otherwise there could be a delay in color development which would result in false negative readings.)

CAUTIONS

Certain drugs may discolor urine and obscure test results. Some common urine-discoloring medicines are listed below.

MEDICINES	*URINE COLOR*
acetaminophen (DATRIL, TYLENOL, etc.)	pink-red
amitriptyline (AMITIL, ELAVIL, etc.)	blue-green
anticoagulants (see section 34)	pink to red to brown
indomethacin (INDOCIN)	green
methyldopa (ALDOMET)	red, darkens on standing
metronidazole (FLAGYL)	dark brown
nitrofurantoin (CYANTIN, MACRODANTIN)	brown, yellow
phenazopyridine (AZODINE, PHENAZ- ODINE, PYRODINE, etc.)	orange to red
phenothiazines (THORAZINE, PROLIXIN, COMPAZINE, MELLARIL, etc.)	pink, red, purple, orange, rust
phenytoin (DILANTIN, etc.)	pink, red, red-brown
rifampin (RIFADIN)	red-orange
salicylates (*aspirin*, EMPIRIN, BUFFERIN, etc.)	pink to red to brown

MEDICINES	*URINE COLOR*
sulfonamides (GANTANOL, BACTRIM, SEPTRA, etc.)	rust, yellow, or brown
triamterene (DYRENIUM)	green, blue with blue fluorescence

142. Eating right to feel better

Eating smaller and more frequent meals is better than eating two or three large ones, but what you eat is even more important.

Fish is particularly good, since it's high in protein and low in fat. In fact, fish liver oil (available in tasteless capsules) is often recommended as a daily vitamin A supplement for diabetics.

> Eat less more often!

Raw foods have aided many diabetics. Dr. John Douglass of the Southern California Permanent Medical Group and Kaiser Foundation Hospital in Los Angeles has found that they can even reduce insulin requirements. He theorizes that raw foods are "less stressful to the human system," and advocates a diet high in raw vegetables, fruits, egg yolks, honey, oils, and goat's milk.

Brewer's yeast can also help a lot—especially if you're a senior citizen. Impaired glucose tolerance is a definite factor in maturity-onset diabetes, and brewer's yeast is a rich source of GTF, the glucose tolerance factor which can potentiate insulin.

Foods rich in vitamins E and C are important. (See section 36 for supplement recommendations.) These are particularly necessary, because diabetics are prone to impeded blood vessels and poor circulation.

143. Any questions about Chapter XX?

Are there any herb teas that are particularly good for diabetics?
There aren't any I know of that will replace insulin, but the leaves of the blueberry plant have been found to lower blood sugar levels. It's recommended that the leaves steep in hot water for half an hour, and that a cup of the tea (always freshly made) be drunk two or three times daily.

CHAPTER XXI

Insomnia is Nothing to Lose Sleep Over

144. Sleep problems of senior citizens

If you're over sixty-five, chances are you actually need less sleep than vigorous, active adults thirty years your junior (though it's not necessarily true that you require much less sleep than you did when you were young). Sleep requirements for older people are around 5 to 7 hours, and women, surprisingly, require more than men.

> Older people often think that they get less sleep than they really do.

The catch is that the older you are the less *continuously* you sleep. Nighttime waking for urination, because of muscle cramps, and so on, frequently causes older people to estimate the amount of sleep they get at much less than it really is. Because of this, many hypnotics and sedatives are often prescribed for senior citizens unnecessarily—especially when some of their sleep problems are simply side effects of medications they're already taking. (See section 56.)

145. Searching for Morpheus over-the-counter can cause trouble

Many people, especially those reluctant to pay for another office visit to the doctor just to discuss insomnia, resort to OTC medications. This can be dangerous, because most OTC sleep-aids contain drugs such as bromides, *aspirin,* or other analgesics, scopolamines, or antihistamines, all of which can have serious side effects (especially for senior citizens), and none of which, except perhaps for antihistamines (which can promote drowsiness), has a rightful place as a sleeping aid.

Though fatal overdoses are rare, sleep-aids can cause mental confusion and memory disturbances, according to a 1979 report issued by the Institute of Medicine. Additionally, antihistamines can repress the stage of sleep associated with dreaming, so that withdrawing from the drug after continued use can temporarily intensify dreams and cause sleep-disturbing nightmares.

146. Why hypnotics aren't hip

Prescription sleeping pills are often quite effective—but they're often quite dangerous, too. (See section 50.)

Though benzodiazepines (VALIUM, DALMANE, ATI-VAN, etc.) are considered safer than barbiturates, the ones that stay in the body for a long time can create potentially serious side effects in the daytime (like diminished driving skills). And because all benzodiazepines are dangerous when combined with alcohol, anyone taking the long-acting variety such as DALMANE should be warned to stay away from liquor for several days after discontinuing the medication.

> Using sleeping pills regularly can make insomnia *worse*!

Most benzodiazepines, though, remain in the system for just

a few hours. What this means is that if your body metabolizes them while you're asleep, you're likely to suffer "rebound insomnia," which may very well be worse than the sleeplessness you had before.

These drugs can depress breathing functions, cause birth defects, aggravate liver disease, and cause problems that will really give you something to lose sleep over. But just in case you aren't convinced, several recent studies have shown that chronic use of these medications only makes insomnia worse!

147. Be an insomnia investigator

Before resorting to medication for occasional difficulties in falling or remaining asleep, why not ask yourself these questions:

- Do I have caffeine late in the evening? (A cola, cup of coffee, or chocolate cake while watching Carson?)
- Have I napped during the day?
- Am I upset about a work or home situation?

If you answered yes to any of the above, you can probably avoid pills and cure your insomnia by a) eliminating the caffeine; b) eliminating the naps; or c) trying to deal with your work or home problems through relaxation techniques and/or therapy.

148. Some natural sleeping potions

Instead of that cup of coffee or drink of coke, give one of the following a try before bedtime:

Nighty-night Shake

1 large banana
¾ cup skim milk
1 tbsp. honey
Blend and drink one hour before bedtime.

Sweet 'n Dreamy

1 cup buttermilk
2 tbsp. honey
juice of 1 lemon
Blend and drink one hour before bedtime.

THE BASICS

- Camomile tea—preferably with milk
                    or simply
- A glass of nice warm milk (it's high in tryptophan—
  and it works!)

See section 54 for additional suggestions.

149. Any questions about Chapter XXI?

Can aspirin help you sleep?
Yes and no. According to researchers at Dartmouth Medical
School in Hanover, New Hampshire, two *aspirins*, which contain
salicylate, can be an effective hypnotic for chronic insomniacs—
but only for a short time. After 2 weeks of use, the *aspirin* loses
much of its sleep-inducing potency.

*My friend told me that there's some sort of sachet that you
can put under your pillow to help you sleep. Do you know
about it?*
It's a folk remedy, but it seems to have worked for a lot of
folks. What you have to do is buy some hops (that's the herb
they use in beer-making) at your local health food shop and
put a handful into a cheesecloth bag. Put the bag inside your
pillowcase and settle down for sweet dreams. The aroma is what's
supposed to "scent" you into dreamland.

Part Six

MIXES THAT DON'T ALWAYS MATCH

CHAPTER XXII

Drugs and Sex

150. What do drugs have to do with your sex life?

A lot! Some of the most widely used drugs can affect the sexual desire and sexual performance of both sexes. In fact some medications, depending on the dosage and the individual, can cause either increased *or* decreased sexual desire and performance.

Patients with a history of sexual problems are most susceptible to these sorts of side effects, but they *can* happen to anyone.

Before you break up your romance or rush to a therapist, why not check with your doctor and the listings that follow and find out if a change in medication is all that's needed to set your libido right?

151. Medicines that can ruin your sex life

These drugs may cause any or all of the following:

- Decreased sexual desire
- Delayed orgasm
- Impotence
- Ejaculation difficulties

DRUG	CATEGORY	SPECIAL NOTES
Amitriptyline (ELAVIL)	antidepressant	
Baclofen (LIORESAL)	muscle relaxant	
Benztropine (COGENTIN)	anticholinergic	
Chlordiazepoxide (LIBRIUM)	tranquilizer/sedative	
Chlorphentermine (PRE-SATE)	amphetamine	especially in women
Chlorthalidone (HYGROTON)	diuretic	
Chlorotrianisene (TACE)	hormone	in men only
Cimetidine (TAGAMET)	ulcer medication	can also lower sperm count
Clofibrate (ATROMID-S)		
Clonidine (CATAPRES)	antihypertensive	
Cyclobenzaprine (FLEXERIL)	muscle relaxant	
Desipramine (NORPRAMIN)	antidepressant	
Dextroamphetamine (AMODEX, BENZEDRINE)	amphetamine	especially in women
Diazepam (VALIUM)	tranquilizer/sedative	
Dienestrol (DIENESTROL CREAM)	hormone	in men only

DRUG	CATEGORY	SPECIAL NOTES
Diethylpropion (TENUATE, TEPANIL)	amphetamine	especially in women
Diethylstilbestrol (DES)	hormone	in men only
Diphenhydramine (BENADRYL, etc.)	antihistamine	
Disopyramide (NORPACE)	antiarrhythmic	
Dydogesterone (DUPHASTON, GYNOREST)	hormone	
Esterfied estrogens (ESTRATAB, EVEX, MENRIUM)	hormone	in men only
Estradiol (ESTRACE)	hormone	in men only
Estrone (MENAGEN)	hormone	in men only
Ethionamide (TRECATOR)	antituberculosis	
Ethisterone	hormone	
Fenfluramine (PONDIMIN)	amphetamine	especially in women
Guanethidine (ISMELIN)	antihypertensive	decreased emission of semen
Hydralazine (APRESOLINE, etc.)	antihypertensive	

DRUG	*CATEGORY*	*SPECIAL NOTES*
Hydrochlorothiazide (HYDRODIURIL)	diuretic	
Hydroxyzine (VISTARIL, ATARAX)	tranquilizer	
Imipramine (TOFRANIL)	antidepressant	
Isocarboxazid (MARPLAN)	antidepressant	
Isopropamide (DARBID)	antispasmodic	
Levodopa (DOPAR, etc.)	antiparkinson	
Lithium (LITHONATE, LITHANE)	antidepressant	
MAO Inhibitors	antidepressant	women may lose ability to achieve orgasm while retaining sexual desire
Meprobamate (EQUANIL, MILTOWN)	tranquilizer/sedative	
Methantheline (BANTHINE)	antispasmodic	
Methyldopa (ALDOMET)	antihypertensive	
Metoprolol (LOPRESSOR)	antihypertensive	
Norethindrone (NORLUTIN)	hormone	

DRUG	CATEGORY	SPECIAL NOTES
Norgestrel (Ovrette)		
Orphenadrine (NORFLEX, etc.)	muscle relaxant	
Oxazepam (SERAX)	tranquilizer/sedative	
Pargyline (EUTONYL)	antidepressant	
Perhexilene (PEXID)	antianginal	
Phenelzine (NARDIL)	antidepressant	
Phenoxybenzamine (DIBENZYLINE)	antihypertensive	
Progesterone (PROGESTA-SERT, PROGESTIN)	hormone	
Propantheline (PRO-BANTHINE)	antispasmodic	
Propranolol (INDERAL, INDERIDE)	antihypertensive	
Protriptyline (VIVACTIL)	antidepressant	
Reserpine (DEMI-REGROTON, DIUPRES, SER-AP-ES, SERPASIL)	antihypertensive	
Spironolactone (ALDACTONE)	diuretic	

DRUG	CATEGORY	SPECIAL NOTES
Thioridazine (MELLARIL)	tranquilizer	causes ejaculatory difficulties without impairing orgasm
Tranylcypromine (PARNATE)	antidepressant	
Trihexyphenidyl (ARTANE)	anticholinergic	

152. Medicines that can heighten sexual arousal

DRUG	CATEGORY	SPECIAL NOTES
Chlordiazepoxide (LIBRIUM)	tranquilizer/sedative	can also cause decreased sexual arousal
Chlorotrianisene (TACE)	hormone	in women only
Danazol (CYCLOMEN, DANOCRINE)	hormone	
Diazepam (VALIUM)	tranquilizer/sedative	can also cause decreased sexual arousal
Dienestrol (DIENESTROL CREAM)	hormone	in women only
Diethylstilbestrol (DES, SYNESTRIN)	hormone	in women only
Esterfied estrogens (ESTRATAB, EVEX, MENRIUM)	hormone	in women only

DRUG	CATEGORY	SPECIAL NOTES
Estradiol (ESTRACE)	hormone	in women only
Estrone (MENAGEN)	hormone	in women only
Ethylestrenol (MAXIBOLIN)	hormone	
Guanethidine (ISMELIN)	antihypertensive	decreases sexual arousal but may cause erotic dreams
Isocarboxazid (MARPLAN)	antidepressants	can also cause delayed orgasm in women and erectile and ejaculation difficulties in men
Meprobamate (EQUANIL, MILTOWN)	tranquilizer/sedative	can also cause decreased sexual arousal
Oxazepam (SERAX)	tranquilizer/sedative	can also cause decreased sexual arousal
Pargyline (EUTONYL)	antidepressant	can also cause delayed orgasm in women and erectile and ejaculation difficulties in men
Phenelzine (NARDIL)	antidepressant	can also cause delayed orgasm in women and erectile and ejaculation difficulties in men

DRUG	CATEGORY	SPECIAL NOTES
Stanozolol (WINSTROL)	hormone	
Testosterone (DELATESTRYL)	hormone	
Tranylcypromine (PARNATE)	antidepressant	can also cause delayed orgasm in women and erectile and ejaculation difficulties in men

153. Drugs and fertility

One of the more recent discoveries about drugs is that they can raise and lower sperm counts. For instance, PERGONAL (*menotropins*), a hormonal medication usually prescribed to treat menopausal and fertility difficulties in women, is now being used on men to increase their sperm count. The drug must be injected intramuscularly 2 to 3 times a week for at least 4 months to produce a significant increase. (Unfortunately, one of the drug's side effects is enlargement of male breasts.)

Many more drugs, though, can *lower* sperm counts. Among them are:

- AZULFIDINE (*sulfasalazine*)—an anti-infective usually used to help control diseases such as enteritis or colitis
- BACTRIM, SEPTRA (*sulfamethoxazole* and *trimethoprim*) —sulfonamides most often prescribed for urinary tract infections
- COLSALIDE IMPROVED (*colchicine*)—an anti-uric acid, antigout drug
- TAGAMET (*cimetidine*)—used often in the treatment of ulcers

154. How to improve your sexuality naturally

The best way to improve your sex drive is to keep your

nutritional status up to par. (See section 64 for a good high energy regimen.)

Vitamin E can increase fertility in males and females, but that it influences the sex drive has yet to be proven, though I have met many happy vitamin-E-takers who are convinced that it does. I have also seen success in cases of impotence with a supplement program of vitamin B_6 and zinc.

Ginseng—though it can't work miracles—has been able to help many men and women improve their sex lives. Taken as a tea or tonic over a period of time, it appears to have a stimulating as well as normalizing effect.

Supplements can help solve sex problems.

Damiana (also known as Turnera) is an herb that has been touted for years as a natural aphrodisiac. It can easily be made into a tea by pouring a cup of boiling water over a teaspoonful of the dried leaves or ¼ teaspoonful of the ground leaf powder. (One to four cups daily is the recommended remedy.)

Probably the most widely known aphrodisiacal herb is sarsaparilla. Most satisfied users of the herb boil one ounce of this root in a pint of water for half an hour and drink wine-sized glassfuls frequently.

And if you're looking for a love potion, the following is alleged to be the best (and tasty, too!):

CUPID'S SPECIAL

½ cup banana (pureed)
½ cup watermelon juice
1 cup papaya juice
1 tsp. ground cloves
Blend and sip slowly.

155. Any questions about Chapter XXII?

Are there any drugs that can cure impotence?
One might be on the market soon. *Yohimbine,* a chemical derived from the tropical African yohimbe tree, is still being

tested by researchers at Queen's University in Kingston, Ontario, but early results have been very promising, especially among men with impotence related to physical problems, like diabetes.

Exactly how the drug helps potency is still unknown, but researchers think that because the chemical blocks—or stimulates—the release of adrenaline at nerve endings in different parts of the body, this action either changes blood flow or the transmission of nerve impulses to genital tissue.

CHAPTER XXIII

Alcohol and Drugs

156. When drinks and drugs don't mix

Almost never! Alcohol can interact adversely with more than one hundred medications. Though your pharmacist or physician might not tell you explicitly not to drink with your medicine, my advice is don't do it unless you've asked and been told that you can.

SOME DRUGS THAT SHOULDN'T MIX WITH ALCOHOL

DRUG	*POSSIBLE EFFECT*
Acetaminophen (TYLENOL, TEMPRA, etc.)	can increase possibility of liver damage and aggravate side effects of drug
Anesthetics	can decrease effectiveness of the onset of anesthesia
Anticoagulants (see section 34)	can decrease or increase anticoagulant effect with dangerous unpredictability

DRUG	*POSSIBLE EFFECT*
Antihistamines (see section 38)	can increase CNS depression and dangerously magnify sedative effects
Aspirin (and all salicylates)	can cause gastrointestinal bleeding and aggravate other side effects of drug
Barbiturates (see section 50)	can increase CNS depression dangerously (often lethally), or with chronic alcohol abuse decrease sedative effect of drug
Benzodiazepines (VALIUM, DALMANE, ATIVAN, SERAX, etc.)	can increase CNS depression dangerously— even for a few days after discontinuing the medication
Bromocriptine (PARLODEL)	can cause nausea and abdominal pain
Chloral hydrate (NOCTEC, ORADRATE, etc.)	can prolong the drug's hypnotic effect
Chloramphenicol (CHLOROMYCETIN)	can cause nausea, abdominal cramps, flushing, and vomiting
Cyloserine (SEROMYCIN)	can cause increased convulsions with chronic alcohol abuse
Diphenoxylate and Atropine (LOMOTIL, etc.)	can increase CNS depression and sedative action
Disulfiram (ANTABUSE)	can cause abdominal cramps, flushing, vomiting, psychotic episodes, confusion

DRUG	POSSIBLE EFFECT
Isoniazid (INH, etc.)	can increase chance of hepatitis, and decrease effect of drug with chronic use of alcohol
Meclizine hydrochloride (ANTIVERT, BONINE, MAREZINE, etc.)	can increase CNS depression and sedative action
Meprobamate (EQUANIL, MILTOWN, etc.)	can increase CNS depression dangerously, or with chronic alcohol abuse decrease sedative effects
Metronidazole (FLAGYL)	can cause nausea, vomiting, abdominal cramps, headache
Narcotics (any and all)	can increase CNS depression dangerously (often lethally)
Phenothiazines (PROLIXIN, COMPAZINE, MELLARIL, VESPRIN, etc.)	can increase CNS depression dangerously
Phenytoin (DILANTIN, etc.)	can decrease anticonvulsant effect with chronic alcohol use and increase anticonvulsant effect with alcohol intoxication
Propranolol (INDERAL)	can mask tachycardia and tremors of alcoholic hypoglycemia

157. Ground zero combinations

Though alcohol can interact adversely with almost all drugs, there are some combinations that are more potentially lethal than others—and these *cannot* be ignored.

DEFINITELY DO NOT DRINK ALCOHOL WITH . . .

- MAO (monoamine oxidase) Inhibitors (MARPLAN, NARDIL, and PARNATE)
- *Methaqualone* (MEQUIN, PAREST, QUAALUDE)
- Barbiturates (AMYTAL, BUTICAPS, BUTISOL, SOMBU-LEX, MEBERAL, GEMONIL, NEMBUTAL, SEDA-DROPS, SK-PHENOBARBITAL, SOLFOTON, SEC-ONAL, TUINAL, LOTUSATE)
- Benzodiazepines (ATIVAN, DALMANE, LIBRIUM, SERAX, VALIUM)
- Tricyclic antidepressants (AMITID, AMITRIL, ELA-VIL, ENDEP, NORPRAMIN, PERTOFRANE, ADAPIN, SINEQUAN, IMAVATE, JANIMINE, SK-PRAMINE, TOFRANIL, AVENTYL, PAMELOR, VIVACTIL, SUR-MONTIL)
- *Codeine*
- *Propoxyphene* (DARVON, DOLENE, PROXAGESIC, PROXENE, SK-65)
- *Meperidine* (DEMEROL, PETHADOL)
- *Disulfiram* (ANTABUSE)
- Any tranquilizer, sedative, hypnotic, or narcotic medication

158. Watch out for those time-release pills

Any drug that's available in time-release or spansule form can become dangerous if taken in conjunction with alcohol. The coating that's supposed to allow the drug to be released slowly over an extended time period (usually 8–12 hours) can dissolve rapidly in alcohol and give you an uncomfortable and potentially toxic dose of the medication.

159. That cup of coffee won't help

The common assumption that coffee—or any other central nervous system (CNS) stimulant—will sober you up, is false. In the first place, the effects of combining caffeine or amphet-amines with alcohol are unpredictable. In the second place, these drugs have—at best—a negligible effect on improving driving or any other skills that are impaired by alcohol.

But what is most important, and most frightening, is that recent studies seem to indicate that caffeine may *worsen* the effects of alcohol on alertness, leaving you unaware of your continuing brain impairment!

160. Any questions about Chapter XXIII?

Are there any drugs that can make me not WANT to have a drink?

It looks as if there's one in the works. According to a study done by Dr. Joseph Zabik, a pharmacology professor at Purdue University, *fluxetine* (a drug now being tested as an antidepressant) allows the body to store more serotonin, which—when there is enough of it—creates an aversion to alcohol.

My 65-year-old mother, who's in pretty good health, a nonsmoker, and really only a moderate drinker, has breathing difficulties when she sleeps. My husband says that it's her two or three "nightcaps" which cause it. Could this be the reason?

There's a very good chance that it is, though you should still check with a doctor, since breathing difficulties are nothing to trifle with—ever! But researchers have found a strong connection between sleep apnea (periods during sleep when breathing stops) and alcohol.

The families of patients with sleep apnea have found that episodes of breath stoppage are worse when the patient has had even just a few drinks. They've also found that the alcohol contributed to more frequent and longer-lasting attacks. (Alcohol consumption also contributes to snoring.) I'd suggest your mother get a good medical checkup—and then try her on some nice warm milk before retiring. It's a much safer sleep-inducer than alcohol.

CHAPTER XXIV

Smoking and Drugs

161. How cigarette smoking affects your medication

All smokers know that smoking is hazardous to their health; most know that it frequently causes disability and death; and some know that it's responsible for one out of every three deaths due to coronary heart disease (to say nothing of cancer). But few smokers are aware that their habit can directly affect their medication. Yet it can—and does!

> If you smoke more than a pack a day, you might be getting less of your medicine than you think!

Smoking speeds up the drug metabolizing enzymes in the liver and accelerates the body's metabolism of the drug. What this does, in essence, is reduce the blood levels and therefore the therapeutic effects of the drug involved.

There is a definite correlation between the amount of cigarettes smoked daily and the extent of the interaction. And anyone who smokes more than 20 cigarettes daily will be more prone to interactions with drugs than someone who smokes fewer cigarettes per day.

162. Those perilous puffs: Drugs that can be affected by smoking

- ASCORBIC ACID—Every cigarette you smoke destroys about 25 mg. to 100 mg. of vitamin C (ascorbic acid), so it's no wonder that smokers tend to have lower serum ascorbic acid levels. But since vitamin C plays a primary role in the formation of collagen, which is important for the growth and repair of body tissue cells, gums, blood vessels, bones, and teeth, this is no mean deficiency.
- BENZODIAZEPINES—These drugs, which include VALIUM, DALMANE, ATIVAN, and SERAX, and which are often prescribed for insomnia, have been found to be less effective for smokers. The more cigarettes a patient smokes, the less likely it is that drowsiness will occur.
- HEPARIN—Smokers have a more rapid elimination of this anticoagulant than nonsmokers.
- INDERAL (*propranolol*)—Smoking has been shown to re duce propranolol levels in the blood, particularly in younger patients. And in the treatment of angina pectoris, smoking inhibits the desired therapeutic effect of INDERAL.
- LASIX (*furosemide*)—Nicotine can reduce the diuretic properties of this drug in laboratory animals. Human studies are still in progress. (See section 40.)
- ORAL CONTRACEPTIVES—Smoking can increase the risk of stroke, myocardial infarction, and thromboembolism, especially in women over 35 years of age who smoke more than 15 cigarettes per day. (See section 49.)
- PHENOTHIAZINES—These drugs, which include THORAZINE, PROLIXIN, COMPAZINE, MELLARIL, VESPRIN, and others, and which are usually prescribed for tranquilizing purposes, have been found to produce less sedative effects in smokers than in nonsmokers.
- PROPOXYPHENE—This analgesic (see section 32) has been rated ineffective in 20 percent of patients who smoke more than a pack of cigarettes daily.

- TALWIN (*pentazocine*)—Smokers who use this as a substitute for nitrous oxide anesthesia, especially during dental surgery, require larger doses than nonsmokers in order for it to be effective.
- THEOPHYLLINE—Increased liver metabolism of this drug in smokers has been shown to shorten its effectiveness as a bronchodilator.
- TRICYCLIC ANTIDEPRESSANTS—(See section 35.) Smokers have been shown to have lower plasma levels of these medications, and these decreased levels are substantial enough to reduce the drug's desired effects. (If you smoke you might need a higher dosage than you're getting.)

163. Smoking and sickness

Is there a connection? You bet there is! Cigarette smoking can

- cause chronic bronchitis and emphysema
- cause cancer of the lung, larynx, mouth, esophagus, bladder, kidney, and pancreas
- interact adversely with oral contraceptives to increase the probability of coronary and cerebrovascular disease
- cause coronary heart disease
- increase the risk of spontaneous abortion and prenatal death
- retard fetal growth, lower birth weight of infants, impair growth and development during early childhood
- worsen symptoms of respiratory and cardiovascular disease
- increase the risk of lung cancer among nonsmokers exposed to cigarette smoke
- change the way many drugs are metabolized in the body

164. Vitamins that can help smokers

As far as I'm concerned, smokers need all the nutritional help they can get, especially from antioxidants such as vitamins A, C, E, and selenium. (Antioxidants neutralize the destructive radical oxygen molecules, such as ozone, carbon monoxide, and so on, in cigarette smoke.) The following regimen is no substitute for quitting, but it can give your body a fighting chance for health.

High-potency multiple vitamins with chelated minerals (time-release preferred)	A.M. & P.M. (with meals)
High-potency chelated multiple mineral	A.M. & P.M. (with meals)
Vitamin C	1,000–2,000 mg., 1 to 3 times daily
Vitamin E	400–1,000 IU daily
Selenium	50 mcg. 1 to 3 times daily
Vitamin A	10,000 IU daily (take for 5 days, then stop for 2)

165. What you should know about quitting

> Nicotine provides the brain with a barrier against unpleasant external stimuli.

It's not easy to stop smoking, and your body knows it. The craving for nicotine is real. Recent studies have shown that nicotine provides a stimulus barrier that protects the brain from unpleasant or distracting external stimuli. In other words, it acts as sort of a buffer for things like annoying noises, arguments, overstimulation of any kind. When you quit smoking, your brain no longer has its nicotine buffer, and external stimuli come charging at you with an unpleasant reality that's greater than if you'd never smoked at all—hence, withdrawal symptoms.

But there's good news in the offing for smokers who want to break the habit without giving up nicotine. A nicotine chewing gum is now available OTC in Switzerland, and by prescription in Canada (NICORETTE). Each stick contains approximately 2–4 mg. of nicotine, and one pack of gum (15 sticks) is said to replace a pack of twenty cigarettes.

In the meantime, since the gum is not yet available in the United States, you can ease the irritability of withdrawal by taking 1 tryptophan (667 mg.) tablet 3 times a day, along with a vitamin B-complex, 100 mg., and vitamin C, 1,000 mg. 1 to 3 times daily. A good high-potency multiple vitamin with chelated minerals should also be taken with breakfast and dinner.

166. Any questions about Chapter XXIV?

My husband smokes, but I don't. Is it true that just the smoke from his cigarettes can really affect me?

It certainly *is* true. As a matter of fact, the smoke which comes from burning tobacco has more carcinogenic tars than inhaled smoke.

If you can't get your husband to quit, I'd suggest you fortify yourself with antioxidants (see section 164) and get yourself a good home air-filter.

Are there any natural ways to unhook me from cigarettes?

Raw, unsalted shelled sunflower seeds will decrease the acidity of the bloodstream in smokers, thus lessening the loss of nicotine. By chewing the seeds, you'll find that you won't want to light up as often—and it will supply the oral gratification by giving your mouth something to do.

CHAPTER XXV

Summing Up

167. How to locate a nutritionally-oriented doctor

For a list of nutritionally-oriented practitioners in your area, write to the following organizations. Be sure to enclose a stamped, self-addressed envelope.

International College of Applied Nutrition
Box 386
La Habra, California 90631

International Academy of Preventative Medicine
10950 Grandview, Suite 469
Overland Park, Kansas 66210

International Academy of Metabiology, Inc.
P.O. Box 15157
Las Cruces, New Mexico 88001

Prevention Magazine Readers' Service
Emmaus, Pennsylvania 18049

Consulting Nutritionists in Private Practice
P.O. Box 345
Cold Springs, New York 10515

American Academy of Medical Preventics
8383 Wilshire Blvd., Suite 922
Beverly Hills, California 90211

American Holistic Medical Association
6932 Little River Tpk.
Annandale, Virginia 22003

168. What to do if you do too much—Poison Control Centers

If you suspect that you or a member of your family has taken an overdose of a medication, contact your doctor or local poison control center immediately!

Poison control centers provide round-the-clock information concerning treatment or prevention of accidents involving poisonous or potentially poisonous substances.

To find out the phone number and address of the Poison Control Center in your area, look in the front of your phone book or write to the Director, National Clearinghouse for Poison Control Centers, Food and Drug Administration, U.S. Department of Health, Education, and Welfare, Bethesda, Maryland 20016—or phone (202) 496-7691. In Canada, contact the Chief of Poison Control Division, Health and Welfare Canada, Ottawa, Ontario K 1A 188.

It's important to have your local Poison Control Center number on hand *before* an emergency arises—and it's wise to keep that number right near your telephone.

AFTERWORD

Great strides in medicine and pharmacology are being made daily, but the same is happening in the field of nutrition. There is no one substance, be it nutrient or drug, that can provide optimal health. But it is my dream that as more and more is learned about the interrelated chemical mysteries of our bodies, doctors will begin to take a more holistic approach to medicine, treating individuals as whole entities, as opposed to simply ministering to individual parts. By so doing, they—as well as the millions who now rely so heavily on drugs—will realize the amazing role vitamins and minerals play in curative as well as preventive medicine.

In the meanwhile, I hope that *The Pill Bible* has given you a better understanding of the medicines you do take, the reasons why you're taking them, and enough information about the drawbacks, cautions, and alternatives to your treatment to intelligently consider and discuss it with your doctor. But, even more, I hope the book has provided you with all you need to know to feel well while getting well. If I've succeeded, your continued good health will be my finest reward.

Dr. Earl L. Mindell

Beverly Hills, California
November 22, 1983

GLOSSARY

Absorption The process by which nutrients are passed into the bloodstream.

Acetate A derivative of acetic acid.

Acetic acid Used as a synthetic flavoring agent, one of the first food additives (vinegar is approximately 4 to 6 percent acetic acid); it is found naturally in cheese, coffee, grapes, peaches, raspberries, and strawberries; Generally Recognized As Safe (GRAS) when used only in packaging.

Acetone A colorless solvent for fat, oils, and waxes, which is obtained by fermentation (inhalation can irritate lungs, and large amounts have a narcotic effect).

Acid A water-soluble substance with sour taste.

Addiction Compulsive use of habit-forming drugs.

Adrenal gland A triangular-shaped gland near each kidney that synthesizes and stores dopamine, norepinephrine, and epinephrine.

Adrenals The glands, located above each kidney, that manufacture adrenaline.

Alkali An acid-neutralizing substance (sodium bicarbonate is an alkali used for excess acidity in foods).

Allergen A substance that causes an allergy.

Allergy Abnormal sensitivity to any substance.

Amino acid chelates Chelated minerals that have been produced by many of the same processes nature uses to chelate minerals in the body; in the digestive tract, nature surrounds the elemental minerals with amino acid, permitting them to be absorbed into the bloodstream.

Amino acids The organic compounds from which proteins are constructed; there are twenty-two known amino acids, but only nine are indispensable nutrients for man—histidine, isoleucine, leucine, lysine, total S-containing amino acids, total aromatic amino acids, threonine, tryptophan, and valine.

Amnesia Memory loss.

Analgesic Drug used to relieve pain.

Anemia Reduction in normal amount of red blood cells.

Aneurysm Localized abnormal dilation of a blood vessel; may be due to congenital defect or weakness of blood vessel wall.

Angina pectoris Severe attacks of pain about the heart, caused by an insufficient supply of blood to the heart.

Anopsia Defective vision, usually from disuse of eye because of muscle weakness, cataract, or refractive errors.

Anorectic Having no appetite.

Anorexia Loss of appetite.

Anorexia nervosa A symptom of mental disturbance which causes loss of appetite for food and compulsive dieting.

Anoxia Insufficient oxygen supply.

Antibiotic Any of various substances that are effective in inhibiting or destroying bacteria.

Anticoagulant Something that delays or prevents blood-clotting; blood-thinner.

Antidyskinetics Drugs used in the treatment of Parkinson's disease.

Antiemetic Remedy to prevent vomiting.

Antigen Any substance not normally present in the body that stimulates the body to produce antibodies.

Antihistamine A drug used to reduce effects associated with colds and allergies.

Antineoplastics Drugs that prevent growth and development of malignant cells.

Antioxidant A substance that can protect another substance from oxidation; added to foods to keep oxygen from changing the food's color.

Antitoxin An antibody formed in response to—and capable of—neutralizing a poison of biologic origin.

APC Aspirin (acetylsalicylic acid), phenacetin, and caffeine; common combination of ingredients in a variety of cold remedies and analgesics.

Aphrodisiac An agent which produces sexual desire.

Apnea Temporary cessation of breathing, usually during sleep.

Arthritis Inflammation of joints.

Asepsis Condition of being sterile, free from germs.

Aspirin Acetylsalicylic acid, used to relieve headaches, pain, fever, and inflammation.

Assimilation The process whereby nutrients are used by the body and changed into living tissue.

Asthma Condition of lungs characterized by decrease in diameter of some air passages; a spasm of the bronchial tubes or swelling of their mucous membranes.

Ataxia Loss of coordinated movement.

ATP A molecule called adenosine triphosphate, the fuel of life, a nucleotide—building block of nucleic acid—that produces biological energy with B_1, B_2, B_3, and pantothenic acid.

Avidin A protein in egg white capable of inactivating biotin.

Bariatrician A weight-control doctor.

Bell's palsy Paralysis of the facial nerve, shown in the weakness of one side of the face.

Beta-adrenergic blocking agent A substance which blocks the transmission of stimuli thereby slowing down the rate of nerve response in the heart, and the heart rhythm itself.

"Beta-blocker" See beta-adrenergic blocking agent.

BHA Butylated hydroxyanisole; a preservative and antioxidant used in many products; insoluble in water; can be toxic to the kidneys.

BHT Butylated hydroxytoluene; a solid, white crystalline antioxidant used to retard spoilage of many foods; can be more toxic to the kidney than its nearly identical chemical cousin BHA.

Bioflavonoids Usually from orange and lemon rinds, these citrus-flavored compounds needed to maintain healthy blood-vessel walls are widely available in plants, citrus fruits, and rose hips; known as vitamin P-complex.

Bradycardia Slow heart rate.

Calciferol A colorless, odorless crystalline material, insoluble in water; soluble in fats; a synthetic form of vitamin D made by irradiating ergosterol with ultraviolet light.

Calcium gluconate An organic form of calcium.

Capillary A minute blood vessel, one of many that connect the arteries and veins.

Carcinogen A cancer-causing substance.

Cardiac arrhythmia Irregular heart action caused by disturbances in discharge of cardiac impulses.

Cardiovascular Pertaining to heart and blood vessels.

Carotene An orange-yellow pigment occurring in many plants and capable of being converted into vitamin A in the body.

Casein The protein in milk that has become the standard by which protein quality is measured.

Catabolism The metabolic change of nutrients or complex substances into simpler compounds, accompanied by a release of energy.

Catalyst A substance that modifies, especially increases, the rate of chemical reaction without being consumed or changed in the process.

Cataract Clouding of the lens of the eye which prevents clear vision.

Catatonia Type of schizophrenia characterized by immobility.

Chelation A process by which mineral substances are changed into easily digestible form.

Chronic Of long duration; continuing; constant.

Cirrhosis A chronic liver disease characterized by dense or hardened connective tissue, degenerative changes or alteration in structure.

CNS Central nervous system.

Coenzyme The major portion, though nonprotein, part of an enzyme; usually a B vitamin.

Cold sores Lesions particularly in and around the mouth caused by herpes simplex virus.

Colitis Inflammation of large intestine.

Collagen The primary organic constituent of bone, cartilage, and connective tissue (becomes gelatin through boiling).

Coma Complete loss of consciousness.

Congenital Condition existing at birth, not hereditary.

Corticosteroid Any of various steroid substances obtained from the adrenal gland.

Corticosterone An adrenal cortex hormone that influences the metabolism of carbohydrates, potassium, and sodium; essential for normal absorption of glucose.

Dehydration A condition resulting from an excessive loss of water from the body.

Delirium Mental disturbance resulting in disorientation, confusion, and excitement.

Dermatitis An inflammation of the skin; a rash.

Desiccated Dried; preserved by removing moisture.

Dicalcium phosphate A filler used in pills which is derived from purified mineral rocks and is an excellent source of calcium and phosphorus.

Diluents Fillers; inert material added to tablets to increase their bulk in order to make them a practical size for compression.

Diuretic Increases flow of urine from the body.

DNA Deoxyribonucleic acid; the nucleic acid in chromosomes that is part of the chemical basis for hereditary characteristics.

Dopamine A compound which increases blood pressure.

Dyspepsia Indigestion.

Dysuria Painful urination.

Edema Excessive accumulation of tissue fluid.

Endogenous Produced from within the body.

Enteric coated A tablet coated so that it dissolves in the intestine, not in the stomach (which is acid).

Enteritis Inflammation of the intestines, particularly the small intestines.

Enuresis Bed-wetting.

Enzyme A protein substance found in living cells that brings about chemical changes; necessary for digestion of food.

Epilepsy Convulsive disorder.

Epinephrine Produced by the adrenal medulla and other tissues, it has also been synthesized and is used as a vasoconstrictor, heart stimulant, and to relieve asthmatic attacks.

Estrogens Female sex hormones.

Excipient Any inert substance used as a dilutant or vehicle for a drug.

Exogenous Derived or developed from external causes.

FDA Food and Drug Administration.

Fibrin An insoluble protein that forms the necessary fibrous network in the coagulation of blood.

Free radicals Highly reactive chemical fragments that can produce an irritation of artery walls, start the arteriosclerotic process if vitamin E is not present; generally harmful.

Fructose A natural sugar occurring in fruits and honey; called fruit sugar; often used as a preservative for foodstuffs and an intravenous nutrient.

Galactosemia A hereditary disorder in which milk becomes toxic as food.

Gallstones Stone-like objects found in gall bladder and its drainage system.

Glaucoma Disease of the eyes in which the pressure of the fluid in the eye increases.

Glucose Blood sugar; a product of the body's assimilation of carbohydrates and a major source of energy.

Glutamic acid An amino acid present in all complete proteins; usually manufactured from vegetable protein; used as a salt substitute and a flavor-intensifying agent.

Glutamine An amino acid that constitutes, with glucose, the major nourishment used by the nervous system.

Gluten A mixture of two proteins—gliadin and glutenin—present in wheat, rye, oats, and barley.

Glycogen The body's chief storage carbohydrate, primarily in the liver.

Gout Upset in metabolism of uric acid, causing inflammation of joints particularly in the knee or foot.

GRAS Generally Recognized As Safe; a list established by Congress to cover substances added to food.

Half-life The time it takes for half the amount of a drug to be metabolized or inactivated (disappear from the bloodstream) by the body (an important consideration for determining the amount and frequency of drug dosage).

Hallucination False perception having no relation to reality and not accounted for by any exterior stimuli; may involve one, all, or any combination of the senses.

Hepatitis Inflammation of liver.

Hesperidin Part of the C-complex.

Holistic treatment Treatment of the whole person.

Homeostasis The body's physiological equilibrium.

Hormone A substance formed in endocrine organs and transported by body fluids to activate other specifically receptive organs.

Humectant A substance that is used to preserve the moisture content of materials.

Hydrochloric acid A normally acidic part of the body's gastric juice.

Hydrolyzed Put into water-soluble form.

Hydrolyzed protein chelate Water-soluble and chelated for easy assimilation.

Hypertension High blood pressure.

Hypervitaminosis A condition caused by an excessive ingestion of vitamins.

Hypoglycemia Low blood sugar.

Hypotension Low blood pressure.

Hypovitaminosis A deficiency disease owing to an absence of vitamins in the diet.

Ichthyosis A condition characterized by a scaliness on the outer layer of skin.

Idiopathic Describes a condition whose causes are not yet known.

Immune Protected against disease.

Infectious Liable to be transmitted by infection.

Inflammation Changes that occur in living tissues when invaded by germs; swelling, pain, heat.

Insulin The hormone, secreted by the pancreas, concerned with the metabolism of sugar in the body.

IU International Units.

Jaundice Increase in bile pigment in blood, causing yellow tinge to skin, membranes, and eyes; can be caused by disease of liver, gallbladder, bile system, or blood.

Lactating Producing milk.

Lactation Secretion of milk by breasts.

Laxative A substance that stimulates evacuation of the bowels.

Linoleic acid One of the polyunsaturated fats, a constituent of lecithin; known as vitamin F; indispensable for life, and must be obtained from foods.

Lipid A fat or fatty substance.

Lipofuscin Age pigment in cells.

Lipotropic Preventing abnormal or excessive accumulation of fat in the liver.

MAO Inhibitors Abbreviation for monoamine oxidase inhibitors; a group of antidepressants that promotes an elevation of levels of amine messengers in the emotional regions of the brain.

Megavitamin therapy Treatment of illness with massive amounts of vitamins.

Menopause Age at which normal cessation of monthly period occurs, usually between 45 and 50.

Metabolize To undergo change by physical and chemical processes.

Narcotic A central nervous system depressant which, in moderate doses, relieves pain and produces sleep; in large doses it can produce unconsciousness or even death; can be addicting.

Nausea Stomach discomfort with the feeling of a need to vomit.

Nitrites Used as fixatives in cured meats; can combine with natural stomach and food chemicals to cause dangerous cancer-causing agents called nitrosamines.

Norepinephrine A hormone produced by the adrenal medulla, similar to epinephrine, and used chiefly as a vasoconstrictor.

Obesity Excessive stoutness.

Ophthalmic Pertaining to eyes.

Ophthalmia Inflammation of eye.

Orthomolecular The right molecule used for the right treatment; doctors who practice preventive medicine and use vitamin therapies are known as orthomolecular physicians.

OSHA Occupational Safety and Health Administration.

Oxalates Organic chemicals found in certain foods, especially spinach, which can combine with calcium to form calcium oxalate, an insoluble chemical the body cannot use.

PABA Para-aminobenzoic acid; a member of the B-complex.

Palmitate Water-solublized vitamin A.

Parasite Any animal or plant which lives inside or on the body of another animal or plant.

Peptic Pertaining to digestive tract.

Photosensitivity Sensitivity to light.

PKU (phenylketonuria) A hereditary disease caused by the lack of an enzyme needed to convert an essential amino acid (phenylalanine) into a form usable by the body; can cause mental retardation unless detected early.

Polyunsaturated fats Highly nonsaturated fats from vegetable sources; tend to lower blood cholesterol.

Predigested protein Protein that has been processed for fast assimilation and can go directly to the bloodstream.

Provitamin A vitamin precursor; a chemical substance necessary to produce a vitamin.

Psychosis Type of insanity in which one loses almost complete touch with reality.

PUFA Polyunsaturated fatty acid.

RDA Recommended Dietary Allowances as established by the Food and Nutrition Board, National Academy of Sciences, National Research Council.

Rhinitis Inflammation of the lining of the nose.

RNA Ribonucleic acid.

Rose hips A rich source of vitamin C; the nodule underneath the bud of a rose called a hip, in which the plant produces the vitamin C we extract.

Rutin A substance extracted from buckwheat; part of the C complex.

Saturated fatty acids Usually solid at room temperature; higher proportions found in foods from animal sources; tend to raise blood cholesterol levels.

Sequestrant A substance that absorbs ions and prevents changes that would affect flavor, texture, and color of food; used for water softening.

Soporific Producing sleep.

Syncope Brief loss of consciousness; fainting.

Synergistic The action of two or more substances to produce an effect that neither alone could accomplish.

Synthetic Produced artificially.

Systemic Pertaining to the whole body.

Tachycardia Rapid beating of heart coming on in sudden attacks.

Teratogen Anything which causes the development of abnormalities in an embryo.

Tocopherols The group of compounds (alpha, beta, delta, epsilon, eta, gamma, and zeta) that make vitamin E; obtained through vacuum distillation of edible vegetable oils.

Toxicity The quality or condition of being poisonous, harmful, or destructive.

Toxin An organic poison produced in living or dead organisms.

Tremor Shake or quiver.

Triglycerides Fatty substances in the blood.

Ulcer Sore or lesion on skin surface or internal mucous membranes.

Unsaturated fatty acids Most often liquid at room temperature; primarily found in vegetable fats.

Urticaria Skin eruptions which are associated with severe itching; hives.

USAN United States Adopted Names Council; cosponsored by the American Pharmaceutical Association (APhA), the American Medical Association (AMA), and the United States Pharmacopia (USP) for the specific purpose of coining suitable, acceptable, nonproprietary names in the drug field.

USRDA United States Recommended Daily Allowances.

Vasodilator A drug which dilates (widens) blood vessels.

Xerosis A condition of dryness.

Zein Protein from corn.

Zyme A fermenting substance.

BIBLIOGRAPHY AND RECOMMENDED READING

It almost goes without saying that a book of this scope could not have been written without the myriad studies and research of numerous doctors, pharmacists, nutritionists, scientists, and other dedicated professionals, to whom I am indebted, whose work in the fields of medicine, pharmacology, and nutrition has not only been the foundation of my knowledge, but enabled me to bring this project, long close to my heart, to fruition.

The following list is given to show my deep and sincere appreciation. Many of the books are highly technical, but others, which I've marked with an asterisk, I wholeheartedly recommend to all concerned individuals for further reading and a way to a more enlightened and healthier future.

*Abrahamson, E. M., and Pezet, A. W. *Body, Mind and Sugar.* New York: Avon Books, 1977.

*Adams, Ruth. *The Complete Home Guide to All the Vitamins.* New York: Larchmont Books, 1972.

*Adams, Ruth, and Murray, Frank. *Minerals: Kill or Cure.* New York: Larchmont Books, 1976.

*Airola, Paavo. *Hypoglycemia, A Better Approach.* Phoenix, AZ: Health Plus, 1977.

American National Red Cross. *Blood: The River of Life.* Washington, DC: 1976.

*Bailey, Hubert. *Vitamin E: Your Key to a Healthy Heart.* New York: ARC Books, 1964, 1966.

*Berkow, Robert, ed. *The Merck Manual.* 14th ed. Rahway, NJ: Merck and Co., 1982.

Bieri, John G. "Fat-soluble vitamins in the eighth revision of the Recommended Dietary Allowances." *Journal of the American Dietetic Association* 64 (February 1974).

Billups, Norman F. *American Drug Index 1982.* Philadelphia: J. B. Lippincott Company, 1982.

*Blau, Sheldon Paul, and Schultz, Dodi. *Arthritis.* New York: Doubleday, 1973.

*Bond, C. Y.; Dobbin, E. V.; Gofman, H. F.; Jones, H. C.; and Lyon, L. *The Low Fat, Low Cholesterol Diet.* New York: Doubleday, 1971.

*Borsaak, Henry. *Vitamins: What They Are and How They Can Benefit You.* New York: Pyramid Books, 1971.

*Brace, Edward R. *The Pediatric Guide to Drugs and Vitamins.* New York: Dell, 1982.

*Bricklin, Mark. *Practical Encyclopedia of Natural Healing.* Emmaus, PA: Rodale Press, 1976.

Brody, Jane E. "Cancer-blocking Agents Found in Foods." *The New York Times,* 6 March 1979.

*Burack, Richard, with Fox, Fred J. *New Handbook of Prescription Drugs.* Revised. New York: Ballantine Books, 1980.

*Burns, David D. *Feeling Good, The New Mood Therapy.* New York: New American Library, 1980.

Burton, Benjamin. *Human Nutrition.* 3rd ed. New York: McGraw-Hill, 1976.

*Cammer, Leonard. *Up From Depression.* New York: Pocket Books, 1969.

*Clark, Linda. *Know Your Nutrition.* New Canaan, CT: Keats Publishing Co., 1973.

*———. *Secrets of Health and Beauty.* New York: Jove Publications, 1977.

Consumer Reports 38. "The U.S. Food and Drug Administration: On Food and Drugs." March 1973.

Consumer Reports. "How Nutritious Are Fast Food Meals?" May 1975.

Consumer Reports 43. "Too Much Sugar." March 1978.

Consumer Reports, Editors of. *The Medicine Show.* Mount Vernon, NY: Consumers Union, 1981.

Cumulative Index for Journal of Applied Nutrition. La Habra, CA: International College of Applied Nutrition, 1947–76, 1976.

*Davis, Adelle. *Let's Eat Right To Keep Fit.* New York: Harcourt, Brace and World, 1954.

*———. *Let's Get Well.* New York: Harcourt, Brace and World, 1965.

*———. *Let's Have Healthy Children.* 2nd ed. New York: Harcourt, Brace and World, 1959.

*de Baïracli Levy, Juliette. *Common Herbs for Natural Health.* New York: Schocken Books, 1974.

Deckert, Robert. "Ant Bites Relieve Arthritis." *Omni,* February 1983.

*DiCyan, Erwin, and Hessman, Lawrence. *Without Prescription*. New York: Simon & Schuster, 1972.

The Drug Abuse Survey Project. *Dealing with Drug Abuse*. A Report to the Ford Foundation. New York: Praeger, 1972.

*Dufty, William. *Sugar Blues*. Philadelphia: Chilton Book Company, 1975.

*Ebon, Martin. *Which Vitamins Do You Need?* New York: Bantam Books, 1974.

*Evens, Wayne O., and Cole, Jonathan O. *Your Medicine Chest*. Boston: Little, Brown & Co., 1978.

Flynn, Margaret A. "The Cholesterol Controversy." *Journal of the American Pharmacy*, NS18 (May 1978).

"Food Facts Talk Back." *Journal of the American Dietetic Association*, 1977.

*Frank, Benjamin S. *No-Aging Diet*. New York: Dial, 1976.

*Fredericks, Carlton. *Eating Right for You*. New York: Grosset and Dunlap, 1972.

*———. *Look Younger/Feel Healthier*. New York: Grosset and Dunlap, 1977.

*———. *Psycho Nutrients*. New York: Grosset and Dunlap, 1976.

*Gomez, Joan, and Gerch, Marvin J. *Dictionary of Symptoms*. New York: Bantam Books, 1972.

Goodhart, Robert S., and Shills, Maurice E. *Modern Nutrition in Health and Disease*. 5th ed. Philadelphia: Lea and Febiger, 1973.

*Graedon, Joe. *The People's Pharmacy*. New York: St. Martin's Press, 1976.

*———. *The People's Pharmacy*. Vol 2. New York: Avon Books, 1980.

Harper, Alfred E. "Recommended Dietary Allowances: Are They What We Think They Are?" *Journal of the American Dietetic Association* 64 (February 1974).

Howe, Phyllis S. *Basic Nutrition in Health and Disease*. 6th ed. Philadelphia: W. B. Saunders Co., 1976.

*Hunter, B. T. *The Natural Foods Primer*. New York: Simon & Schuster, 1972.

International College of Applied Nutrition. *Journal of Applied Nutrition*. La Habra, CA: 1974–1976.

International College of Applied Nutrition. *Nutrition—Applied Personally*. La Habra, CA: 1978.

International Nutritional Anemia Consultative Group (INACG). *Guidelines for the Eradication of Iron Deficiency Anemia*. New York: 1976.

International Vitamin A Consultative Group (IVACG). *Guidelines for the Eradication of Vitamin A Deficiency and Xerophthalmia*. New York: 1976.

Journal of the American Dietetic Association. "Vitamin-Mineral Safety, Toxicity, and Misuse." 1978.

Katz, Marcella. *Vitamins, Food, and Your Health*. Public Affairs Committee, 1971, 1975.

*Kordel, L. *Health Through Nutrition.* New York: MacFadden-Bartell, 1971.

Krupp, M. A., and Chatton, M. J. *Current Medical Diagnosis and Treatment.* Los Altos: Long Medical Publications, 1982.

LaPlace, John. *Health.* New York: Appleton-Century-Crofts, 1972.

*Linde, Shirley. *The Whole Health Catalog.* New York: Rawson Associates Publishers, 1977.

*Lucas, Richard. *Nature's Medicines.* New York: Prentice-Hall, 1966.

*Lust, John. *The Herb Book.* New York: Bantam Books, 1974.

"Marijuana: The Health Questions." *Consumer Reports* 40 (March 1975).

*Martin, Alice A., and Tenenbaum, Frances. *Diet Against Disease.* Boston: Houghton Mifflin, 1980.

*Martin, Clement G. *Low Blood Sugar: The Hidden Menace of Hypoglycemia.* New York: Arco Publishing Co., 1976.

Martin, Marvin. *Great Vitamin Mystery.* Rosemont, IL: National Dairy Council, 1978.

*Mason, David, and Dyller, Fran. *Pharmaceutical Dictionary and Reference for Prescription Drugs.* New York: Playboy Paperbacks, 1981.

*Mayer, Jean. *A Diet for Living.* New York: David McKay, 1975.

Medical Economics. *Physician's Desk Reference.* 36th ed. Oradell, NJ: Medical Economics Company, 1982.

Mitchell, Helen S. "Recommended Dietary Allowances Up to Date." *Journal of the American Dietetic Association* 64 (February 1974).

National Dairy Council. Nutrition Source Book, Rosemont, IL: 1978.

National Health Federation Bulletin. November 1978.

National Nutrition Consortium, American Dietetic Association. *Nutrition Labeling: How It Can Work For You.* 1975.

National Nutrition Education Clearing House. *Nutrition Information Resources for the Whole Family.* 1978.

National Research Council. *Recommended Dietary Allowances.* 8th ed., revised. Washington, DC: National Academy of Sciences, 1974.

National Research Council. *Toxicants Occurring Naturally in Foods.* 2nd ed. Washington, DC: National Academy of Sciences, 1973.

*Newbold, H. L. *Dr. Newbold's Revolutionary New Discovery About Weight Loss.* New York: Rawson Associates Publishers, 1977.

*———. *Mega-Nutrients for Your Nerves.* New York: Peter H. Wyden, 1978.

New York State Medical Society Drug Abuse Committee. *Desk Reference on Drug Misuse and Abuse.* New York, 1981.

*Null, Gary and Steve. *The Complete Book of Nutrition.* New York: Dell, 1972.

Nutrition Almanac. New York: McGraw-Hill, 1973.

Nutrition Foundation. *Index of Nutrition Education Materials.* Washington, DC: 1977.

Nutrition Foundation, Inc. "Present Knowledge in Nutrition." *Nutrition Reviews.* 1976.

*Panos, Maesimund, and Heimlich, Jane. *Homeopathic Medicine at Home.*

Los Angeles: J. P. Tarcher, 1980. Distributed by Houghton Mifflin Co., Boston.

*Passwater, Richard A. *Super Nutrition.* New York: Dial, 1975.

*Pauling, Linus. *Vitamin C and the Common Cold.* New York: Bantam Books, 1971.

*Pearson, Durk, and Shaw, Sandy. *Good News for Smokers.* Huntington Beach, CA: The International Institute of Natural Health Sciences, Inc., 1980.

*Phillips, Joël L., and Wynne, Ronald D. *Cocaine: The Mystique and the Reality.* New York: Avon Books, 1980.

*Poe, William D. *The Old Person in Your Home.* New York: Scribner's, 1969.

*Pomeranz, Virginia E., and Schultz, Dodi. *The Mothers' and Fathers' Medical Encyclopedia.* New York: New American Library, 1977.

*Pritikin, Nathan. *The Pritikin Permanent Weight-Loss Manual.* New York: Grosset and Dunlap, 1981.

*Rodale, J. I. *The Complete Book of Minerals for Health.* 4th ed. Emmaus, PA: Rodale Books, 1976.

*——. *The Encyclopedia of Common Diseases.* Emmaus, PA: Rodale Press, 1976.

Roe, Daphne A. *Handbook: Interactions of Selected Drugs and Nutrients in Patients.* Chicago: The American Dietetic Association, 1982.

*Rosenberg, Harold, and Feldzaman, A. N. *Doctor's Book of Vitamin Therapy: Megavitamins for Health.* New York: Putnam, 1974.

*Rubinstein, Morton K. *A Doctor's Guide to Non-Prescription Drugs.* New York: New American Library, 1977.

*Ruthe, Eshleman, and Winston, Mary, comps. *The American Heart Association Cookbook.* New York: Ballantine, 1973.

*Samuels, Mike, and Bennett, Hal. *The Well Body Book.* New York: Random House, 1973.

*Seaman, Barbara and Gideon. *Women and the Crisis in Sex Hormones.* New York: Rawson Associates Publishers, 1977.

*Sehnert, Keith W., with Eisenberg, Howard. *How To Be Your Own Doctor.* New York: Grosset and Dunlap, 1975.

*Shute, Wilfrid E., and Taub, Harold J. *Vitamin E for Ailing and Healthy Hearts.* New York: Pyramid Books, 1969.

*Silverman, Harold M., and Simon, Gilbert I. *The Pill Book.* 2nd ed. New York: Bantam Books, 1982.

*Spock, Benjamin. *Baby and Child Care.* New York: Simon & Schuster, 1976.

Thomas, Clayton L., ed. *Tabers Cyclopedic Medical Dictionary.* 13th ed. Philadelphia: F. A. Davis, 1977.

Underwood, Eric J. *Trace Elements in Human and Animal Nutrition.* 4th ed. New York: Academic Press, 1977.

United Nations. Food and Agriculture Organization. *Calorie Requirements,* 1957, 1972.

U.S. Department of Agriculture. *Amino Acid Content of Food,* by M. L. Orr and B. K. Watt, 1957; rev. 1968.

U.S. Department of Agriculture, Consumer and Food Economics Institute, Agricultural Research Service. *Composition of Foods: Raw, Processed, Prepared,* by Bernice K. Watt and Annabel L. Merrill, 1975.

U.S. Department of Agriculture. *Energy Value of Foods: Basis and Derivation,* by Annabel L. Merrill and Bernice K. Watt, 1973.

U.S. Department of Agriculture. *Nutritive Value of American Foods* by Catherine F. Adams, 1975.

U.S. Department of Health, Education and Welfare. *Consumer Health Education: A Directory,* 1975.

U.S. Department of Health, Education and Welfare. *Ten-State Nutrition Survey.* Washington, DC: U.S. Government Printing Office, 1968–70.

The United States Pharmacopeial Convention. *The Physicians' and Pharmacists' Guide to Your Medicines.* New York: Ballantine, 1981.

U.S. President's Council on Physical Fitness and Sports. *Exercise and Weight Control,* by Robert E. Johnson. Urbana, IL: University of Illinois Press, 1967.

U.S. Senate. Select Committee on Nutrition and Human Needs. *Diet and Killer Diseases with Press Reaction and Additional Information.* Washington, DC: U.S. Government Printing Office, 1977.

U.S. Senate. Select Committee on Nutrition and Human Needs. *National Nutrition Policy: Nutrition and the Consumer II.* Washington, DC: U.S. Government Printing Office, 1974.

*Wade, Carlson. *Health Tonics, Elixirs and Potions for the Look and Feel of Youth.* West Nyack, NY: Parker Publishing Company, 1971.

*——. *Magic Minerals.* West Nyack, NY: Parker Publishing Company, 1967.

*——. Miracle Protein. West Nyack, NY: Parker Publishing Company, 1975.

*——. *Vitamin E: The Rejuvenation Vitamin.* New York: Award Books, 1970.

Williams, Roger J. *Nutrition Against Disease.* New York: Pitman Publishers, 1971.

*Winter, Ruth. *A Consumer's Dictionary of Food Additives.* New York: Crown, 1978.

*Wolfe, Sidney M., and Coley, Christopher M. *Pills That Don't Work.* New York: Farrar, Straus & Giroux, 1980.

*Young, Klein, Beyer. *Recreational Drugs.* New York: Berkley, 1982.

*Yudkin, John. *Sweet and Dangerous.* New York: Peter H. Wyden, 1972.

Index of Drugs
(brand and generic names)

Note: Brand names have initial letter capitalized; generic names are in lower-case *italic*.
Types of drugs (e.g., antihistamines) will be found in the General Index.

General Index

Note: This index includes general references to classes or types of drugs; for particular brand or generic names, see the Index of Drugs.

Allergies:
　to drugs, 29–30, 36–40
　　analgesics, 59
　　antibiotics, 36, 37, 39, 64
　　mechanism of, 36
　　regimen for, 38
　and nasal decongestants, 27
　regimen for congestion relief
　　in, 27
　See also Antihistamines
Aloe vera, 242
Alpha amylase, 202
Amebiasis, 230
Amebicides, 43
American Academy of Medical
　Preventics, 310
American Heart Association, 275
American Holistic Medicine
　Association, 310
American Medical Association
　(AMA), 201, 204
American Society of Bariatric
　Physicians, 101
Amino acids, 168, 201
Aminosalicylates, 149
Amphetamines, 5, 148, 201, 208
　abuse of, 212–14
　barbiturates with, 215
　and birth defects, 100
　and heat stroke, 155
　in pregnancy, 179
　as weight reducers, 199, 200,
　　204
Analeptic agents, 43
Analgesics (pain relievers), 44,
　55–60
　and antidiarrheals, 76
　and antihistamines, 79
　cautions on, 58–59
　food interactions of, 58
　injection of, 22
　natural replacements for,
　　59–60
　side effects of, 38, 56–60
　tranquilizers with, 123, 124
　uses of, 55–56
Anaphylactic shock, 36–37
Anesthetic drugs, 44
　alcohol with, 299
　inhalational, and heat stroke,
　　155
Angina, *see* Antianginals;
　Cardiovascular preparations

Anorexics, *see* Appetite
　suppressants
Antacids, 44
　and anticoagulants, 68
　drug interactions of, 246–47
　and Lanoxin (digoxin), 249
　and laxatives, 112
　phosphate depletion by, 196
　in pregnancy, 178
　sodium in, 268
　replacement of nutrients
　　depleted by, 162
　sugar-free, 191–92
　and tranquilizers, 124
Anthelmintics, 44
Antialcohol preparations, 44
Antianginals, 21, 44, 45
　See also Cardiovascular
　　preparations
Antiarrhythmics, 44, 45
Antiarthritics, 44, 86–89, 258–59
　and aspirin, 248
　cautions on, 88, 89
　food interactions of, 88
　natural, 89
　side effects of, 87–88, 146, 147,
　　149, 150, 258–59
Antiasthmatics, 22
　sugar-free, 192
Antibacterials, 44
Antibiotics, 60–66
　amebicidal, 43
　allergies to, 36, 37, 39, 64
　and anti-uric acid drugs, 97
　brand names of, 9
　cautions on, 64–65
　and children, 189–90
　definition of, 44
　and dairy products, 26
　dosage of, 20
　in elderly, 255–56
　food interactions of, 64, 65
　and fruit juice, 26, 64, 65
　injection of, 22
　and lactation, 197–98
　and laxatives, 112
　natural replacements for, 65
　pick-me-up for, 160
　side effects of, 61–64, 76,
　　189–90
　storage of, 15, 16
　sugar-free, 192
　uses of, 60–61, 66

Barbiturates (*con't.*)
  allergies to, 36, 37
  amphetamines with, 215
  and analgesics, 58
  and antidiarrheals, 76
  and antihistamines, 79
  cautions on, 122–24
  defense against theft of
    nutrients by, 163
  food interactions of, 122
  with "heavy" narcotics, 221
  natural alternatives to, 123–24
  side effects of, 118, 146, 148,
    150, 151
  uses of, 118
Basil tea, 136
Benzodiazepines, 118–22, 180, 209,
  212, 305
  alcohol with, 300, 302
  commonly abused, 213
  for insomnia, 283–84
  side effects of, 150, 152,
    283–84
  and smoking, 305
  and Tagamet, 125
Best-selling drugs, 47–53
Beta-adrenergic blocking agents,
  45, 102, 104, 106, 129, 247
  side effects of, 147, 150, 151
  See also Cardiovascular
    preparations
Bioavailability, 9
Biofeedback techniques, 267,
  274
Biologicals, 45
Biotin (coenzyme R; vitamin H):
  as analgesic, 59
  best sources of, 142
  and muscle pain, 89
Birth control, *see* Oral
  contraceptives
Birth defects:
  and amphetamines, 100
  and Bendectin, 91
  and caffeine, 31
  and Pill, 176
  and topical hydrocortisone,
    179
  and tranquilizers/sedatives, 180
Blood clots:
  and Pill, 115, 175
  and vitamins, 68, 105
  See also Anticoagulants

Blood diseases:
  and anticholinergics/
    antispasmodics, 94
  and anti-uric acid drugs, 97
Blood sugar:
  and drugs, 277–78
  See also Diabetes; Urine sugar test
Blood-thinning drugs, *see*
  Anticoagulants
Blueberry tea, 281
Brand-name drugs, generic drugs
  vs., 8–9
Breast cancer, Pill and, 176
Breastfeeding, *see* Lactation
Brewer's yeast, 138
  and diabetes, 73, 280
  and levodopa, 18–19
  and reproductive system, 115
Bronchial dilators, 45, 126–27
  sugar-free, 192
Bronchitis:
  and antidiarrheals, 76
  and smoking, 306
Bulk producers, 200
Burns, aloe vera and, 242

Cabbage juice, 95
Cade, Robert, 266
Caffeine, 31–33
  and alcohol, 302–3
  amounts contained in beverages
    and chocolate (table), 33
  amounts contained in drugs
    (table), 32–33
  and antibiotics, 64
  and appetite suppressants, 100
  and bronchial dilators, 126, 127
  defense against theft of
    nutrients by, 163
  dependence on, 210, 211
  and heart disease, 274
  and hemorrhoids, 255
  and high blood pressure, 267
  and hot weather, 155
  and insomnia, 284
  and iron deficiency, 19
  and MAO inhibitors, 70
  during pregnancy, 31
Calciferol, *see* Vitamin D
Calcium, 71
  and amphetamine abuse, 214
  best sources of, 144
  and conjunctivitis, 129